SPINAL DEFORMITIES
AND NEUROLOGICAL DYSFUNCTION

SEMINARS IN NEUROLOGICAL SURGERY SERIES

Pediatric Neurological Surgery
Edited by Marc. S. O'Brien

Spinal Deformities and Neurological Dysfunction
Edited by Shelley N. Chou and Edward L. Seljeskog

Surgery of the Posterior Fossa
Edited by William Buchheit and Raymond Truex, Jr.

Neural Trauma
Edited by Robert Bourke

Spinal Deformities and Neurological Dysfunction

Sponsored by the Subcommittee on Continuing Education II (Expanded Program), American Association of Neurological Surgeons and Congress of Neurological Surgeons

Editors:

Shelley N. Chou,
M.D., Ph.D.
Professor and Head
Department of Neurosurgery
University of Minnesota
Medical School
Minneapolis, Minnesota 55455

Edward L. Seljeskog,
M.D., Ph.D.
Professor
Department of Neurosurgery
University of Minnesota
Medical School
Minneapolis, Minnesota 55455

Raven Press ▪ New York

Raven Press, 1140 Avenue of the Americas, New York, New York 10036

Made in the United States of America

Library of Congress Cataloging in Publication Data
Main entry under title:

Spinal deformities and neurological dysfunction.

(Seminars in neurological surgery series)
Includes bibliographical references and index.
1. Spine—Abnormalities.   2. Spine—Wounds and
injuries.   3. Spinal cord—Abnormalities.   4. Spinal
cord—Wounds and injuries.   I. Chou, Shelley N.
II. Seljeskog, Edward L.   III. Series.
 DNLM: 1. Spinal diseases.   2. Spine—Abnormalities.
3. Neurologic manifestations.   4. Spinal injuries.
WE725 S7592
RD768.S65   617'.375   78-3009
ISBN 0-89004-183-0

Preface

This volume provides a review of the group of diseases of the spine generally referred to as the spinal deformities. It presents the current state of our understanding of the nature and progression of these conditions, and discusses their management. Sections deal with both basic and clinical information relating to embryological, developmental, diagnostic, and therapeutic aspects of spinal deformities, with or without neurological dysfunction.

Because these diseases are not among the most common and are most often slowly progressive, only a limited number of physicians have had, to date, a knowledgeable, therapeutic approach for managing them. In addition, approaches have differed among orthopedic and neurological surgeons, and the need for urological and physiatric input and counseling provides added dimensions to good therapy.

It is hoped that this volume will provide the neurological surgeon, orthopedic surgeon, and neurologist with a better understanding of the spinal deformities and their management.

The Editors

Acknowledgments

The editors would like to express their deep appreciation to the Joint Committee on Continuing Education in Neurosurgery of the American Association of Neurological Surgeons, the Congress of Neurological Surgeons, and the Office of Continuing Medical Education of the Medical School of the University of Minnesota for their support in organizing a symposium on the subject which is the topic of this book. Particularly we would like to express our thanks to Dr. George Tindall who is Chairman of the Committee, and to Dr. Douglas Fenderson of the University of Minnesota, for their encouragement and support in making this project possible.

Contents

Contributors

David S. Bradford, *Department of Orthopaedic Surgery, University of Minnesota Medical School, Minneapolis, Minnesota 55455*

Shelley N. Chou, *Department of Neurosurgery, University of Minnesota Medical School, Minneapolis, Minnesota 55455*

Theodore Cole, *Department of Physical Medicine and Rehabilitation, University of Michigan Medical School, Ann Arbor, Michigan 48104*

Donald L. Erickson, *Department of Neurosurgery, University of Minnesota Medical School, Minneapolis, Minnesota 55455*

Lois A. Gillilan, *110 Calle Royale, Santa Fe, New Mexico 87502*

Lawrence Gold, *Department of Radiology, University of Minnesota Medical School, Minneapolis, Minnesota 55455*

John E. Lonstein, *Department of Orthopaedic Surgery, University of Minnesota Medical School, Minneapolis, Minnesota 55455*

Lowell Lutter, *Department of Orthopaedic Surgery, University of Minnesota Medical School, Minneapolis, Minnesota 55455*

James M. Morris, *Department of Orthopaedic Surgery, University of California, San Francisco, California 94143*

Gaylan Rockswold, *Department of Neurosurgery, University of Minnesota Medical School, Minneapolis, Minnesota 55455*

Edward L. Seljeskog, *Department of Neurosurgery, University of Minnesota Medical School, Minneapolis, Minnesota 55455*

E. Shannon Stauffer, *Division of Orthopaedic Surgery and Rehabilitation, Southern Illinois University School of Medicine, Springfield, Illinois 62702*

Roby Thompson, *Department of Orthopaedic Surgery, University of Minnesota Medical School, Minneapolis, Minnesota 55455*

Robert Winter, *Department of Orthopaedic Surgery, University of Minnesota Medical School, Minneapolis, Minnesota, 55455*

Spinal Deformities and Neurological Dysfunction, edited by S. N. Chou and E. L. Seljeskog. Raven Press, New York © 1978.

Embryology of the Spinal Cord and Vertebral Column

John E. Lonstein

Department of Orthopaedic Surgery, University of Minnesota, Minneapolis, Minnesota 55455

Understanding the normal embryology of the vertebral column and spinal cord is necessary before appreciating some of the congenital anomalies that can occur. As events in embryological development occur at the same time, this chapter is divided into three parts: (a) development of the somites, (b) development of the spinal cord, and (c) development of the vertebral column.

DEVELOPMENT OF THE SOMITES

In the earliest stages, the embryonic disc has two layers: ectoderm on the future dorsal aspect with the amniotic cavity on one side, and the endoderm, ventrally forming the roof of the yolk sac (day 12 gestational age). At the cephalad end of the two-layered embryonic disc, the layers are fused, forming the prochordal plate and caudally the ectoderm forms the primitive streak. Just cranial to the primitive streak the cells thicken, forming the primitive knot, or Hensen's node. In the center of this, the cells invaginate to form the primitive pit, which is equivalent to the blastopore of lower animals. From the primitive pit, cells migrate between the ectoderm and endoderm in a cranial direction, forming the notochordal process, which grows to meet the prochordal plate. At the same time, cells migrate from the primitive streak between the ectoderm and endoderm around the notochordal plate cranially, forming the third embryonic layer, the mesoderm (day 18). The primitive pit deepens into the solid notochordal process, which now becomes tubular. The notochordal process fuses with the endoderm in the roof of the yolk sac, and these layers degenerate so that the upper half of the notochordal process comes to lie directly in contact with the yolk sac forming a ridge in the roof of the yolk sac, the notochordal plate. At this stage, there is thus a direct communication between the yolk sac and amniotic cavity through the notochordal process and the primitive pit. The exact stage and site of closure of the primitive pit and disappearance of Hensen's node are unknown. This connection is called the neurenteric canal. The endoderm on each side of the notochordal plate curl under until they meet and reunite, producing the true notochord. This process starts cranially and extends caudally, and is completed by the end of 4 weeks (4 mm; 25 somite stage). The presence of the true notochord induces the thickening in the overlying ectoderm to form the neural plate (see below).

When the notochord and neural tube develop, the intraembryonic mesoderm lies as a complete layer between the ectoderm and endoderm. This mesoderm thickens to form two longitudinal paramedian columns, the paraxial mesoderm. Laterally the mesoderm differentiates into the intermediate mesoderm and lateral mesodermal plate. The intermediate mesoderm gives rise to the genitourinary system, and the lateral mesodermal plate is continuous with the mesoderm of the somatopleure lining the amniotic cavity and the splanchnopleure lining the yolk sac.

Starting on the 20th day of gestation, the cells of the paraxial mesoderm undergo a segmentation process, forming the somites, which are separated by intersegmental fissures. The first cranial somites appear in the middle portion of the embryo just caudal to the cranial end of the notochord. Because of the predominant cephalic development following this stage, the region where the first somites appear actually corresponds to the future occipital area. This segmentation process proceeds in a craniocaudal direction, and at the end of the fifth week 42 somites are formed in the human embryo. On the external surface of the embryo, these somites are visible as a series of elevated beads along the dorsolateral surface of the embryo. On cross section, the somites are wedge-shaped with a central cavity, the myocele.

During this somite stage, the older cranial somites show some internal specialization. The cells lying dorsolateral to the myocele plus the cells that are proliferating in this primitive cavity form the skin integuments. The more medial cells form the dorsal musculature. These cells migrate between the endoderm and the ectoderm, forming the paravertebral muscles, and combine with the somatopleure, forming the muscles of the limbs and the abdominal wall. The ventromedial cell mass forms the sclerotome. These cells migrate medially toward the neural tube and notocord, forming the vertebral column (see below) (2,5,10).

SPINAL CORD EMBRYOLOGY

There are three stages of the spinal cord development (4): (a) Neurulation is involved in formation of the majority of the spinal cord and the brain cranially; (b) canalization; and (c) retrogressive differentiation. The latter two apply only to the caudal end of the neural tube.

Neurulation

At approximately the 17th to 19th day, the first differentiation toward formation of a nervous system occurs. The midline cells of the ectoderm (neural plate) are specialized as neurectoderm and the process of neurulation separates these cells from the amniotic cavity forming a complete covering of ectoderm. The neural plate sinks inward, becoming grooved, and its lateral margins curl over to join in the dorsal midline to form the neural tube. This tube is probably formed by a migration of cells in this area. The first fusion of the folds occurs at the 6 to 7 somite stage, the site of initial fusion being at the level of the third or fourth somite. The folding process proceeds cranially and caudally, forming a closed tube with cranial and caudal openings (Fig. 1). These openings are the anterior and posterior neuropores. The cells at the junction of the neural plate and ectoderm are specialized and become detached from both the neural tube and the ectoderm, forming a mass of cells lying on the dorsal side of the neural tube, the neural crest. These cells are specialized and form the dorsal spinal ganglion cells.

Approximately 3 days after the neural tubes begin to fuse, the cranial portion of the neural tube differentiates to form the brain. With this marked proliferation of cells the embryo flexes, forming the cephalic flexure accentuated by the downgrowth of the hypothalamic region. The neural folds continue to close rostally; the site of final closure is called the anterior neuropore. This is located at the most rostal portion of the neural groove,

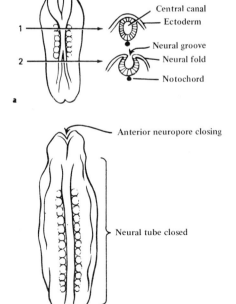

Central canal
Ectoderm
Neural groove
Neural fold
Notochord

Anterior neuropore closing

Neural tube closed

Posterior neuropore open
(closes in Stage XII)

FIG. 1. a: Neurulation. Dorsal view of an embryo at 22 days' gestation during initial fusion of the neural folds. On the right side are cross sections taken at the level of arrows 1 and 2. **b:** Dorsal view at 24 days' gestation. A large part of the neural tube has closed. The anterior neuropore closes at this stage and the posterior neuropore closes 2 days later. (From ref. 4.)

which corresponds to the lamina terminalis in older embryos. This occurs at the 13 to 20 somite stage at approximately 24 days; the central canal of the neural tube is now continuous with the amniotic cavity through the posterior neuropore.

The posterior neuropore closes 2 days later on the 26th day at the 21 to 29 somite stage. The average time of closure is probably at the 25 somite stage. This would locate the site of closure at approximately the first or second lumbar vertebra with variations of two or more segments cranially or caudally, i.e., T11 to L4. When the posterior neuropore closes, the initial stage of neural tube formation is complete with the internal cavities of the nervous system completely sealed. The communication between the central canal and the amniotic cavity is now absent.

Canalization

With the complete closure of the neural tube, the low lumbar, sacral, and coccygeal segments have not developed. The differentiation in this area is less well described when compared to the process of neuralization. Recent studies suggest the process to be similar to that which occurs in birds consisting of canalization of the caudal cell mass and retrogressive differentiation.

At the caudal end of the neural tube and notocord, there is a large aggregate of undifferentiated cells extending into the primitive tail fold. At this stage the only structures in this region are the mesonephros and hindgut. Some of the undifferentiated cells near the end of the neural tube orient themselves around small vacuoles (days 22–32). These undifferentiated cells around the vacuoles attain the appearance of ependymal cells. The vacuoles coalesce, and when this occurs two or three layers of cells take on the appearance of neural cells. These coalescing vacuoles make contact with the central canal of the neural tubes just cranially, and this results in elongation of the neural tube into the tail (Fig. 2) (3,4). Studies on embryos

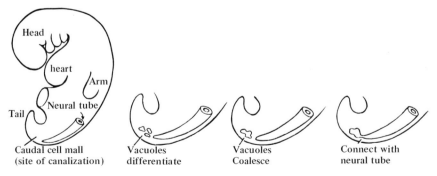

FIG. 2. Canalization as a possible factor in elongation of the neural tube after closure of the posterior neuropore. (From ref. 4.)

at this stage of development show that the process of canalization lacks the precise changes of neurulation.

Retrogressive Differentiation

At this stage, there is regression and degeneration of the structures formed during the canalization phase. This occurs in a precise manner and thus is not a degenerative process; it was termed "retrogressive differentiation" by Streeter (7–9).

Initial retrogressive differentiation occurs at the 11 mm stage with disappearance of the embryonic tail. The regression of the neural tubes starts later at the 13- to 18-mm stage (48 days). The changes in the neural tube involve changes in the vertebral structures at the same time. With the retrogressive differentiation, three structures are derived from the embryonic neural tube: ventriculus terminalis, filum terminale, and the coccygeal medullary vestige (Fig. 3). The lumen of the central canal decreases in size in its middle portion. The ventriculus terminalis remains throughout as an identifiable space. This is found in most cases within that portion of the spinal cord which will become the conus medullaris, and occasionally it is found in upper filum terminale. The level of this space has been identified by Streeter (7) and Kunitomo (3) as occurring opposite the developing 36th vertebra (coccygeal 2). This level obviously forms the distal extent of the definitive spinal cord, and Streeter (7) showed that it starts opposite coccygeal 2 or 3 at the 28-mm stage (i.e., 58 days), opposite S2 at the 67-mm stage (70 days), opposite L5 at the 111-mm stage (95 days), and opposite L2 at the 21-mm stage (160 days). This ascension of the spinal cord is due to the

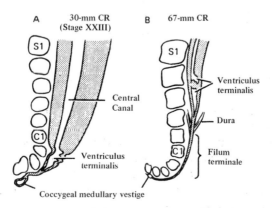

FIG. 3. Relationship of structures involved in the process of retrogressive differentiation. (From ref. 4.)

differential growth that occurs in the embryo between the spinal cord and vertebral column. The vertebral column grows at a faster longitudinal rate than the spinal cord, causing the distal end of the spinal cord to "migrate" cranially. There is controversy as to exactly when the spinal cord reaches its adult position opposite L2 or between L1 and L2, and studies have put this between the embryonic period to the second year of life.

At the 30-mm stage (60 days), the caudal neural tube atrophies leaving a small ependymal rest at the tip of the coccygeal segments. This is known as the coccygeal medullary vestige. Between this vestige and the ventriculus terminalis, the neural tube atrophies into a fibrous band, the filum terminalae. This persists throughout life and is divided into a cranial intradural subarachnoid part and the caudal part fused with the dura.

VERTEBRAL COLUMN FORMATION

Formation of the vertebral column (1,4,5,6) occurs at the 3-mm stage, or 23 days, with the formation of the somites and the sclerotome. As described, the somites are separated by intersegmental fissures, with the medial cells forming the sclerotome. These cells migrate to form the first of three successive vertebral columns. Initially there is formation of mesenchymal vertebral column, which becomes cartilagenous and then osseus.

Membranous Phase

The initial migration of the mesenchyme from the sclerotome is toward the notochord, and it surrounds the notochord as a perichordal sheet. These cells around the notochord contribute to the bodies of the vertebrae and the intervertebral discs. They thus separate the notochord from the endoderm and the neural tube. This process starts initially in the cervical region on the 23rd day at the 3-mm stage and proceeds caudally. During the next 7 to 10 days, cells migrate in a dorsal direction to form the neural arch, and other cells migrate in a ventrolateral direction to form a primordia of the rib. Thus at the end of the membranous stage the cell migration in these three directions from the sclerotome forms the membranous anlage of the definitive vertebral body.

Starting on approximately the 24th day, a resegmentation occurs in the membranous vertebral bodies (Fig. 4). The cells of the somite divide into two cell masses: a cranial (less cellular) and a caudal (more cellular) portion. The division between these two halves is formed by the sclerotomic fissure of von Ebner. At the end of the membranous stage some areas have both intersegmental and sclerotomic fissures. The dense caudal cells of one somite unite with the less-dense cranial cells of the next caudal somite, forming the definitive vertebral body. The cells of the more-dense section

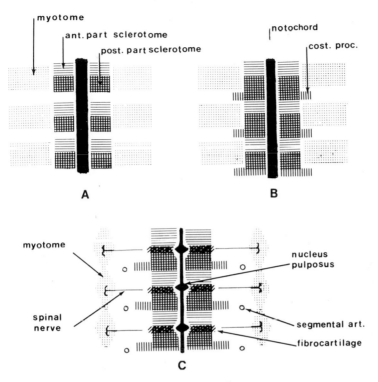

FIG. 4. Development of the vertebrae. **A:** Initial stage of somite formation with a cranial (less cellular) and caudal (more cellular) portion. **B:** Cell migration with intersegmental and sclerotomic fissures shown. **C:** Final stage. (From ref. 5.)

abutting on the sclerotomic fissure contribute the basic cells which form the annulus fibrosis and the enchondral growth plates of a centrum. In addition in the mesechymal stage, the notochord, which up to this time is of uniform thickness, shows a diameter change. The cells in the area of the future centrum become compressed and degenerate, whereas the cells in the area which will become the future intervertebral disc proliferate, forming the nucleus pulposus. Alternately cells may migrate to the future disc region.

It is noted that with this resegmentation process the somite, which was originally segmental with a segmental muscle mass and spinal nerve with a artery lying between the segments, is converted into a definitive segment of the vertebral body. This is actually intersegmental, spanned by the segmental muscle. The embryological segmental spinal nerve now lies in an intersegmental position while the embryological intersegmental vessel comes to lie across the center of the definitive vertebral body. This resegmentation process probably starts in the lower cervical and upper thoracic areas, extending cranially and caudally.

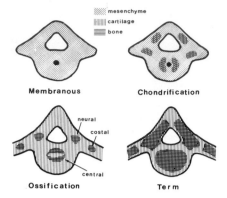

FIG. 5. Development of the vertebrae showing the stages of membranous development, chondrification, and ossification. (From ref. 5.)

Chondrification

From the 40th day of gestation onward (11 to 14 mm), centers of chondrification appear in the mesenchyme of the membranous vertebral column. In the centrum, these centers appear initially on either side of the notochord before fusing. Two centers appear in the neural arches lateral to the neural tube, and their dorsal fusion establishes the neural arch and spinous process. Two additional centers appear at the union of the arch and the centrum, and these extend laterally into the transverse processes. The development of the neural arches starts at a stage later than the centrum as the cells in this area are still proliferating to close the neural arch. The cells dorsal to the neural tube initially have two layers. The outer layer of cells forms the arches by proliferation at the tips of the processes. This proliferation extends dorsally. The inner layer is called the closure membrane, and the inner cells form the dura mater by fusing across the midline, whereas the outer cells are continuous with the outer layer. At approximately the 50-mm crown–rump (CR) length stage, these tips are almost united across the dorsal surface of the spinal cord in the upper cervical region, in contact in the low cervical region and completely fused in the thoracic and lumbar regions.

During the 7th and 8th weeks, the anterior and posterior longitudinal ligaments form from the mesenchymal cells that surround the cartilagenous vertebrae. The relationship to the cartilagenous vertebrae is identical to that in the adult state; the anterior longitudinal ligament is strongly adherent to the anterior surface of the centrum, whereas the posterior longitudinal ligament is attached only to the edge of the disc.

Between the cartilagenous centra, a ring of cells establishes the anulus fibrosis around the portion of the notochord that will become the nucleus pulposus. With further chondrification on the centra the notochord is destroyed in this area and remains in the vertebral disc area. Small remnants of the notochord remain in the centrum despite ossification as the mucoid streak.

Ossification

The stage of ossification overlaps that of chondrification. In the vertebral arches, this process follows a craniocaudal pattern beginning in the cervical and thoracic regions from the 33-mm CR length stage, extending to the sacral region at the 52-cm CR length stage. In the vertebral bodies, the ossification begins in the thoracolumbar region at the same time (at 34-mm CR length) and extends cranially and caudally involving the sacral bodies at about 55 mm CR length and the cervical vertebral bodies at 70 mm CR length.

As with other bones of the skeleton, ossification of the vertebrae involves primary and secondary ossification centers. The primary centers in the vertebral body occur initially anterior and posterior to the vestigeal mucoid streak. These two areas rapidly coalesce to form a center for the centrum, this starting in the low thoracic and upper lumbar region at the 34-mm stage. In the vertebral arches, there are two ossification centers on each side. Although ossification starts in the arches in the cervical region, the laminae of the arches first unite in the lumbar region and this subsequent union progresses cranially.

From the 20th to 24th weeks, enlargement of the ossification center for the centrum divides the vertebral body into two cartilagenous plates with endochondral ossification which face the intervertebral discs. These discs are nourished by vascular tufts from the vertebral body, but the tufts do not extend into the anulus, all the nutrition being derived from diffusion. Around the ventral and lateral periphery of the centrum and disc interface, a C-shaped cartilagenous ring develops to form the ring apophysis, which ossifies during the second postnatal decade. This ring firmly anchors the anulus to the body and, once ossified, receives the Sharpey's fibers of the anulus. Secondary centers of ossification develop during the 15th to 17th years in the tips of the transverse processes and spinous processes plus in the ring apophyses.

It must be remembered that this description applies to the typical vertebra in the thoracic area, the exact site of the ossification centers being modified with specialization of the vertebrae in different areas of the vertebral column; e.g., in the lumbar area there are secondary centers for the mamillary processes. It must be noted that throughout the vertebrae the eventual fusion of the vertebral arches and the centrum occurs well anterior to the pedicles and at the site of the neurocentral synchondrosis. Thus the definitive vertebral body includes more than just the bone derived from the ossific center of the centrum, and the terms vertebral body and centrum are not interchangeable.

REFERENCES

1. Epstein, B. S. (1976): Embryological consideration. In: *The Spine—Radiological Test and Atlas.* Lea & Febiger, Philadelphia.

2. James, C. C. M., and Lassman, L. P. (1972): *Spinal Dysraphism—Spina Bifida Occulta.* Butterworth, London.
3. Kunitomo, K. (1918): The development and reduction of the tail and of the caudal end of the spinal cord. *Contrib. Embryol.,* 18:161–198.
4. Lemire, R. J., Loeser, J. D., Leech, R. W., and Alvord, E. C. (1976): *Normal and Abnormal Development of the Human Nervous System.* Harper & Row, New York.
5. Parke, W. W. (1975): Development of the spine. In: *The Spine,* edited by R. H. Rothman and F. A. Simeone. Saunders, Philadelphia.
6. Sensenig, E. C. (1949): The early development of the human vertebral column. *Contrib. Embryol.,* 33:21–51.
7. Streeter, G. L. (1919): Factors involved in the formation of the filum terminale. *Am. J. Anat.,* 25:1–11.
8. Streeter, G. L. (1942): Developmental horizons in human embryos: Description of age groups 11, 13 to 20 somites and age groups 12, 21 to 29 somites. *Contrib. Embryol.,* 30:211–245.
9. Streeter, G. L. Developmental horizons in human embryos: Description of age groups XIX, XX, XXI, XXII, and XXIII. *Contrib. Embryol.,* 230:167–196.
10. Tuchmann-Duplessis, H., David G., and Haegel, P. (1972): *Illustrated Human Embryology, Vol. I: Embryogenesis.* Springer Verlag, New York.

*Spinal Deformities and Neurological
Dysfunction,* edited by S. N. Chou and E. L.
Seljeskog. Raven Press, New York © 1978.

Vascular Supply of the Spinal Cord: Clinical Significance

Lois A. Gillilan

110 Calle Royale, Santa Fe, New Mexico 87502

The first extensive studies of the blood supply to the human spinal cord were published by Adamkiewicz (2–4) and Kadyi (48,49). These were the only sources of accurate information until Tureen (77), Suh and Alexander (75), and Herren and Alexander (40) described the blood supply 50 years later. Since then most investigators (13,32,63,66,81) have been in essential agreement with the early work. References to the literature are made here only when the information is especially pertinent to this discussion.

The blood supply to the spinal cord of a normal, healthy individual is adequate for its function. There are both anatomic and physiologic factors, however, which can impose critical limitations on the circulation should any interference on either the arterial or venous side occur. Nerve tissue has a span of viability to total anoxia of only 5 to 10 min (22,41,72). The restricted number of feeding (medullary) vessels, together with relatively ineffectual superficial collateral channels, place the spinal cord in a vulnerable situation. The limitations of the anatomic pattern may curtail the circulation of blood and jeopardize the continued functional existence of the neuronal and glial elements with their sensitivity to lack of oxygen. With these considerations in mind, it must be concluded that the spinal cord has a relatively poor blood supply.

Spinal arteries arise from the posterior segmental branches of the descending aorta and from the common iliac, supreme intercostal, ascending, and/or deep cervical and vertebral arteries. An anterior and a posterior radicular ramus begins at each intervertebral foramen and supplies the corresponding nerve root and spinal ganglion. The spinal medullary branches of the spinal arteries, however, are not segmental in the adult but arise asymmetrically. Each one accompanies the nerve root without giving off any branches before joining either the anterior median spinal artery or the posterior arterial plexus.

There are 7 to 10 anterior medullary arteries which supply the anterior two-thirds of the spinal cord (Fig. 1A). One large artery joins the anterior median spinal artery in the region of the cervical enlargement, usually at

11

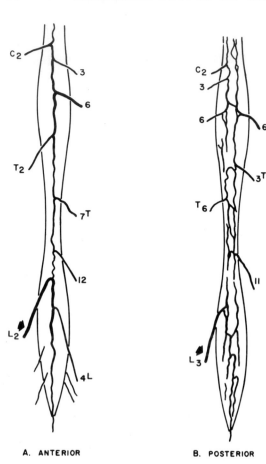

FIG. 1. Composite diagrams made from arterial injections of infant spinal cords. **A:** Eight anterior medullary arteries form the anterior median spinal artery, whose caliber is greatest over the lumbar and cervical enlargements. The major blood supply to the lumbosacral cord is furnished by the great anterior medullary artery (*arrow*). **B:** The superficial arteries on the posterior aspect form bilateral, irregular anastomosing channels with which the posterior medullary arteries unite. The great posterior medullary artery is indicated by the arrow. (From ref. 35.)

A. ANTERIOR   B. POSTERIOR

C5 or C6. This bifurcates into an ascending and a descending limb, each of which then becomes continuous with the segment above and below. There may be one or two, occasionally three, additional cervical medullary arteries. Only the uppermost one or two of these arise(s) from the vertebral artery during its course through the transverse foramina of the cervical vertebrae. Contrary to some statements, the anterior spinal artery formed by the spinal rami of the intracranial portion of the vertebral artery rarely contributes to the anterior median spinal artery. This anastomosis is huge in carnivores, especially in the dog (36), but it is of no significance in man.

The anterior median spinal artery runs the full length of the spinal cord, from the first cervical segment downward over the conus medullaris. It is large in the cervical region, especially over the enlargement. In the thoracic region the anterior median spinal artery tapers from above downward, and by the time it anastomoses with the great anterior medullary artery it may be difficult to see grossly. In this region it receives only two or three medullary arteries. For its length, although possibly not for its total volume, the thoracic cord is the poorest in respect to arterial feeders.

The largest and longest feeding vessel is the great anterior medullary artery (of Adamkiewicz), and it usually accompanies the second lumbar nerve root on the left side, variable between T8 and L4 (32,49,75), in a long course upward. When this vessel reaches the anterior median fissure, its descending limb turns acutely caudally and tapers over the lumbosacral enlargement and filum terminale. This section of the anterior median spinal artery has the largest diameter. Its ascending limb is very small and anastomoses with the thoracic component of the artery. Occasionally another small medullary artery joins the anterior median spinal artery below the great anterior medullary artery.

The posterior third of the spinal cord is supplied from a plexus fed by 12–16 posterior medullary arteries (32,49) (Fig. 1B). Although the posterior plexus is incomplete at times, it still forms an anastomotic system better than the anterior median spinal artery with its variable diameter. A fine, wide-meshed arteriolar pial (coronal) plexus interconnects the posterior network and the anterior median spinal artery, deriving its blood supply from both sources. The diameter of the vessels making up this plexus renders it inadequate for collateral circulation.

INTRINSIC BLOOD SUPPLY

Arteries entering the spinal cord are of two types: (a) the central (sulcal) arteries through which arterial blood flows centrifugally into the gray matter of the anterior and lateral horns and into the adjacent white matter of the anterior two-thirds of the cord; and (b) the centripetal system (2,3,20) of vessels made up of the coronal and posterior plexuses, serving the posterior third of the cord and the peripheral margins of the lateral and anterior white matter (Fig. 2). The central arteries leave the anterior median spinal artery and pass posteriorly through the anterior median fissure, without branching,

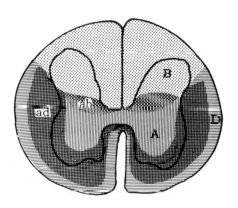

FIG. 2. Distribution of the intrinsic arteries of the spinal cord. (A) Area of distribution of the central artery. (D) Penetrating arteries from the lateral and ventral pial plexus. (ad) Area which may be supplied by either the central or lateral and ventral penetrating arteries (R) Region served by the penetrating arteries from the posterior plexus. (ab) Area which may be covered by either the central or by the posterior penetrating arteries. (From ref. 32.)

and turn alternately to the right or the left (32,35,40,49,77,81). Only rarely do the central arteries bifurcate, reflecting their embryologic origins in paired anterior spinal channels (27,42,44). Although the two channels eventually fuse into a single midline artery, the central arteries retain their laterality.

Adamkiewicz (2,3) counted a total of 250 to 300 central arteries in the adult human spinal cord. The number of central arteries supplying each cord segment varies with the region of the cord. They are most numerous in the lumbosacral enlargement—approximately 34/cm of cord length, according to Woolam and Millen (81)—where they take a nearly horizontal course through the fissure, and the segments supplied are short. In the thoracic region, where the number of central arteries is reduced (14/cm), their posterior course tends to be oblique or even longitudinal. The capillary networks here are spread over a long segment. The vessels in the cervical cord number approximately 24/cm and are intermediate in plane and territory served. It may very well be that the reduced number of central arteries in the thoracic cord and the spreading out of the capillary plexuses are factors which help make the region especially susceptible to reduced oxygen supply.

In the gray matter of the anterior horn, the central arteries branch immediately into precapillaries and capillaries, forming a dense network about the ganglion cells (3,24,32,49,75). There is evidence that, in mammals, nerve cells supplying extensor muscles are more superficial in the anterior horn and that those related to the flexors lie deeper in the gray matter (21,62).

The *intrinsic veins of the spinal cord* do not parallel the arteries but have an anatomic pattern all their own. The earliest reliable description of

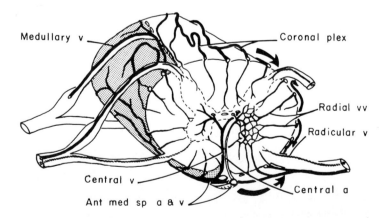

FIG. 3. Cleared preparation of an adult spinal cord in which the veins have been injected. A central artery is illustrated along with the capillary plexus in the anterior horn. A central vein and its tributaries are shown, as are medullary and radicular veins, the formation and disposition of the radial veins, and the coronal venous plexus. (a) Artery, (Ant med sp a & v) Anterior medullary spinal artery and vein. (plex) Plexus. (v) Vein. (vv) Veins. (From ref. 35.)

these veins is that of Kadyi (48,49), followed 50 years later by those of Tureen (77), Alexander and his colleagues (40,75), and Gillilan (34,35). The intrinsic spinal veins comprise two morphologic systems: (a) a central vein or anterior median group, and (b) a radial group (34). The central group is made up of all the central veins and their many branches which empty into the anterior median spinal vein(s). In the region of the anterior white commissure, many venules from both halves of the cord converge in a stellate pattern to form a central vein (Fig. 3). These venules drain the capillary plexuses of the anterior gray and white commissures, the medial cell columns of the anterior horn, and the white matter of the anterior funiculus. Intersegmental anastomoses extend upward and downward in the region of the commissures, and in the anterior median fissure additional anastomoses take place between the central veins themselves. The anterior median spinal vein overlies the fissure, beneath the artery and nearer the mouth of the fissure. Its diameter is not uniform, and it may be double at times. That portion lying caudal to the great anterior medullary vein is of large caliber and tapers downward over the conus medullaris and filum terminale. Draining into this longitudinal system are the central veins and many small, often tortuous tributaries from the adjacent pial venular plexus.

The rest of the spinal cord (i.e., the lateral and posterior white matter, the posterior horns, and the lateral margins of the anterior horns) is drained by the radial vein system. At the periphery of the gray matter short venules arising in the capillary plexus or in the wide-meshed plexus in the white matter join to form the radial veins. They pass toward the surface where they empty into the coronal venous plexus, which has no anatomic relationship with the coronal arteriolar plexus. The posterior veins, in comparison to those on the anterior and lateral surfaces, are large and very tortuous. They tend to be longitudinally oriented over the posterior median sulcus and along the line of entrance of the posterior nerve rootlets. They are more dense over the enlargements.

Venous blood flows through the superficial venous networks toward the medullary veins which accompany certain nerve roots. Blood from the posterior plexus and the posterior half of the lateral plexus leaves through numerous posterior medullary veins (Fig. 4). As the veins of the lateral

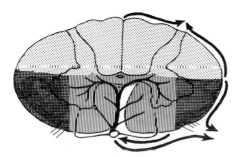

FIG. 4. Intrinsic venous drainage pattern of the spinal cord. The posterior half (*stippled*) is drained through the coronal plexus into the posterior medullary veins. The anterior half (*vertical lines and cross-hatching*) is drained by way of the anterior medullary veins. The medial portion drains through the central vein system into the anterior median spinal vein. Arrows indicate the direction of flow of venous blood. (From ref. 34.)

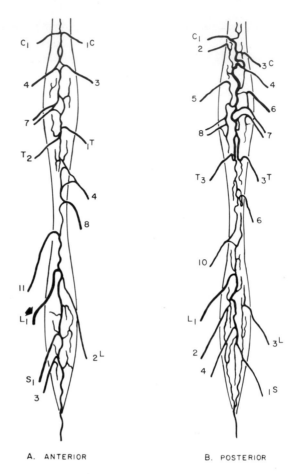

A. ANTERIOR   B. POSTERIOR

FIG. 5. Adult spinal cords in which veins were injected. **A:** The anterior median spinal vein extends longitudinally along the anterior median fissure. Asymmetrical anterior medullary veins, arising mainly from this vessel, drain the anterior segment of the cord. A great anterior medullary vein is indicated by the arrow. **B:** The posterior superficial veins are large and plexiform, and are tortuous over the enlargements. The posterior medullary veins drain the posterior half of the cord and are especially numerous in the cervical region. (From ref. 35.)

coronal plexus converge posteriorly in order to join a posterior medullary vein, they crowd into the narrow angle between the nerve rootlets and the cord itself. Any increase in pressure in this area can be transmitted to the thin-walled venules and interfere with venous drainage from the posterior half of the cord ipsilaterally. Blood from the anterior half of the lateral and the anterior coronal plexuses is carried by 8 to 12 or 14 anterior medullary veins (34,35) (Fig. 5). It should be noted that each nerve root has its own tiny radicular vein. These should not be confused with the medullary veins which drain the spinal cord.

All venous blood, whether from the spinal cord, the meninges, or the epidural plexus, leaves the vertebral canal through the intervertebral vein, or plexus of veins, surrounding the spinal nerve at the intervertebral foramen. These, in turn, communicate with the external (paravertebral) plexus and the cranial dural sinuses, and eventually drain into the abdominal and thoracic cavities through the segmental veins. Inferiorly, the internal and external vertebral plexuses communicate with the pelvic plexus by way of large veins which anastomose with the iliac veins.

PHYSIOLOGY OF THE CIRCULATION OF THE SPINAL CORD

It is not enough to know the anatomic pattern of the arteries supplying the spinal cord. The physiologic principles of circulating blood going to all parts of the cord, especially the gray matter, must also be kept in mind. Heart rate and blood pressure maintain blood flow. The perfusion pressure (the difference between the arterial and venous pressures) must not fluctuate to any degree, and it must remain at a level sufficiently high to meet the metabolic needs of the nervous elements. On the arterial side, should the heart fail and blood pressure fall, delivery of oxygen also falls below the level required to sustain the nerve cells. Should the venous pressure rise inordinately circulation is slowed, and should venous pressure fall there is general circulatory failure.

In a study of the vulnerability of spinal cord structures to anoxia, Gelfan and Tarlov (30) found that cell bodies of neurons are less resistant than interneurons and intramedullary primary afferent neurons. Abrupt onset of anoxia by complete ischemia shortens the survival time of all structures, and signs of dysfunction occur rapidly. The degree of recovery from lack of oxygen is inversely proportional to the length of the anoxic period. In cases where the blood supply is only chronically slowed or is gradually reduced over any length of time, clinical signs are delayed for a period of hours, days, or weeks. Functional loss can result from damage short of anatomic destruction.

In studies carried out on rabbits, dogs, and monkeys, Krogh (55,56) determined that motor cells located at the circumference of the anterior horn are more resistant to ischemia than those at the center. Since there is no difference in the density of the vessels peripherally and centrally, the resistance of the cells does not depend on the abundance of the vessels. Rather, the peripheral cells are nearer the arterial end of the capillaries, and the central cells are nearer the venous end. In the presence of slowed circulation or lowered oxygen tension, the peripheral cells use up the oxygen first, and the central cells are subject to lower oxygen levels. Different species of animals survive anoxia to the central nervous system differently (41). Different individuals of the same species may also respond differently, and it is said that the young of any species are more resistant to anoxia than older individuals.

COLLATERAL CIRCULATION

Underlying the loss of function are two major considerations: (a) (physiologic) the short period of viability of neurons (discussed above); and (b) (anatomic) the lack of effective collateral circulation within the spinal cord itself and to the spinal cord.

Intrinsic Collateral Circulation

The neurons of the central nervous system are supplied by arterioles which go, with few or no branches, directly to a nuclear mass. White matter receives far fewer arterioles and often is supplied only by branches of an arteriole going to a nucleus. The penetrating arterioles terminate in a capillary network, either within a gray mass or in the white matter. The continuity of all capillaries in the spinal cord has been demonstrated (13,40, 66,75,81), and it is now generally conceded that arteries and veins form an unbroken network of capillaries that is continuous throughout the gray and white matter. Because of the small caliber of the intrinsic vessels, the lowered blood pressure, and the decreased rate of flow through the vascular bed (for discussion see ref. 33), the total volume of blood delivered to the neural elements of the spinal cord is not sufficient to meet the nutritional requirements following an ischemic insult that lasts more than a few minutes.

Extrinsic Collateral Circulation with Clinical Correlation

Extravertebral collateral channels to the spinal cord are not particularly good. Most spinal arteries arise from the segmental branches of the aorta and common iliacs, and have a long course from their origins to the intervertebral foramina. Although there are anastomoses with segmental rami above and below, they are usually ineffective. Surgical procedures involving the aorta may and do interfere with the blood supply to the spinal cord by obstructing the flow of blood in one or more medullary artery(ies). Even a bolus of contrast medium administered for abdominal aortography (1,8, 15,25,43,53,57) has been known to interrupt the flow of oxygen long enough to produce paraplegia. Possibly of more interest at present, with attention being directed to cardiac arrest followed by resuscitation, is that spinal cord damage has been reported with the major pathology being located in the caudal region of the cord as an anterior spinal artery syndrome (31).

Occlusion of the arterial blood supply to the anterior two-thirds of the spinal cord results clinically in the typical picture of the anterior spinal artery syndrome (32,54,73). The point of the obstruction may be located anywhere from the anterior median fissure to the aorta. The nearer the occlusion is to the cord, the more circumscribed is the lesion. Involvement of some central arteries or of the anterior median spinal artery produces a transverse lesion with little upward and downward extent. In contrast, extravertebral arterial occlusions result in spinal cord lesions that have considerable upward and downward spread. When a segmental or medullary artery (other than the great anterior medullary artery) is obstructed, the greatest damage is at the level of entrance of the artery, but changes are also seen in the adjacent segments on either side (12,29,66,80,82). There seems to be a "watershed" for adjacent medullary arteries, with the effective area of supply approximately midway between two incoming bloodstreams (23,32).

In the cervical region, however, the potential collateral situation is much better. Branches of the external carotid artery anastomose extensively with each other and have profuse connections across the midline. The vertebral artery is interconnected with the ascending and deep cervical and occipital arteries, and sends branches into the massive arterial plexus within the posterior muscle masses.

Clinical problems involving the cervical cord are many and for the most part result from compression of the spinal cord and its associated structures. The cord itself is relatively immobile in this region, being anchored at the foramen magnum and held in place below by the spinal nerves and the denticulate ligaments. Mechanical compression may be caused by anything that encroaches on the space of the vertebral canal (17,68), be it a ruptured disk (59,74), bony spurs (6,18), ossification of the posterior longitudinal ligament (61), or meninges (52). Epidural lesions such as varicosities of the epidural veins, epidural hemorrhage (64,65), or tumors (metastatic and otherwise) in the epidural space or of the vertebral column (5,14) may also cause cord compression. Whether the compression is exerted directly on the cord or involves blood vessels at the site of the primary impingement, or whether there is secondary pressure on the contralateral side of the cord and/or the arteries has been debated (16,50,69,70,76). Keeping in mind that the arteries have thin walls with little muscle and that they, as well as the intrinsic arterioles and capillaries, are easily compressed, it seems likely that pressure of any force would obstruct some of them, perhaps most of them.

The thoracic and lumbar regions of the spinal cord are subject to the same forces of compression as the cervical cord when the spinal canal is narrowed for essentially the same reasons (79). Ruptured disks often occur in the lower thoracic and lumbar areas. Below the conus medullaris the spinal nerve roots receive the compressive force, and if the great anterior medullary artery is involved the entire lumbosacral enlargement in its anterior two-thirds is affected. A single nerve root is more likely to be involved if the lesion is in the vicinity of the intervertebral foramen. Epstein and Malis (26) state that herniation of an intervertebral disc into a congenitally narrowed spinal canal is not uncommon in achondroplastic dwarfs, causing compression of the spinal cord and cauda equina.

Lateral deformities of the spine (e.g., scoliosis) may result in compression of the structures in the intervertebral foramina on the concave side and stretching of the spinal nerves and their accompanying blood vessels on the convex side. There may be distortion of the cord itself, with or without compression or obstruction of blood vessels.

Involvement of the posterior third of the spinal cord by arterial obstruction seems to be rare. Reasons given for this sparing are the plexiform character of the posterior spinal arteries and the large caliber of the vessels making up the plexus. Hughes (45) reported a case of thrombosis of the posterior spinal arteries following intrathecal injection of phenol for intractable pain with autopsy confirmation. Two additional cases reported by Hughes are inconclusive.

The anatomic patterns of the veins draining the spinal cord were recently described (34,35). However, their clinical involvement has not yet been fully elucidated. These vessels are even more fragile than the arteries because of their extremely thin walls (endothelium covered by adventitia), the low pressure of the blood circulating in them, and the lack of valves (11), except perhaps for valves in the medullary veins at their junction with the vertebral plexus (19). The vertebral veins are subject to all of the problems of veins in general: thrombosis, thrombophlebitis (46), and transport of emboli of all types (7,9), which can be deposited at any level of the body because of the blood currents that ebb and flow depending on the increase or decrease in the pressures in the abdominal and thoracic cavities (10). As suggested earlier, venous obstruction is just as devastating to circulation of blood as arterial obstruction. Hallenbeck et al. (38,39) recently showed that damage to the spinal cord during decompression is the result of accummulation of air bubbles in the epidural veins, which eventually completely block venous return. The lesions in the spinal cord are identical to that described as the spinal vein syndrome by Gillilan (34). This syndrome and its symptom complex of upper motor neuron paraplegia, loss of sphincter control, and sensory dissociation was observed in ascending thrombophlebitis or the epidural ascending spinal paralysis of Spiller (28,37,47,51,58,60, 67,71,78).

SUMMARY

(a) The arterial blood supply to the spinal cord was described. The medullary arteries are limited to 7 to 10 anteriorly and 12 to 16 posteriorly. The superficial coronal plexus is made up of arterioles that are inadequate as collateral channels. Intrinsically there is an all-pervading capillary plexus that is likewise incapable of furnishing collateral circulation.

(b) Venous drainage of the medial aspect of the anterior horns and white matter of the anterior funiculus is good. The remainder of the cord is drained by radial veins into a coronal and posterior plexus which channels blood into anterior and posterior medullary veins. Spinal veins are essentially valveless and belong to the vertebral vein system of Batson. They communicate freely with veins of the head and thoracic and abdominal cavities, and with the pelvic plexus.

(c) The anatomic limitations are further complicated by the fact that nerve tissue has a period of viability from complete anoxia of only 5 to 10 min, a period too short to establish effective collateral circulation. Incomplete anoxia or gradually developing anoxia from ischemia results in varying degrees of cell damage, from depression followed by recovery to complete destruction.

(d) Other than circulatory failure, either arterial or venous, a major cause of vascular lesions in the spinal cord is vessel obstruction. Some clinical examples are discussed.

ACKNOWLEDGMENT

This investigation was supported in part by Public Health Service grant HE-06276 from the Pathology Study Section of the National Heart and Lung Institute.

REFERENCES

1. Adams, H. D., and van Geertruyden, H. H. (1956): Neurologic complications of aortic surgery. *Ann. Surg.,* 144:574–610.
2. Adamkiewicz, A. (1881): Ueber die mikroskopischen Gefässe des menschlichen Rücken-markes. *Trans. Int. Med. Cong.,* 1:155–157.
3. Adamkiewicz, A. (1881): Die Blutgefässe des menschlichen Rückenmarkes. I. Die Ge-fässe der Ruckenmarkssubstanz. *Sitzungsb. Akad. Wissensch. Wien Math.-Naturw. Cl.,* 84:469–502.
4. Adamkiewicz, A. (1882): Die Blutgefässe des menschlichen Rückenmarkes. II. Die Gefässe der Ruckenmarksoberfläche. *Sitzungsb. Akad. Wissensch. Wien Math.-Naturw. Cl.,* 85:101–130.
5. Alexander, E., Jr., Davis, C. H., Jr., and Field, C. H. (1956): Metastatic lesions of the vertebral column causing cord compression. *Neurology (Minneap),* 6:103–107.
6. Allen, K. L. (1952): Neuropathies caused by bony spurs in the cervical spine with special reference to surgical treatment. *J. Neurol. Neurosurg. Psychiatry,* 15:20–36.
7. Anderson, R. (1951): Diodrast studies of the vertebral and cranial venous system to show their probable role in cerebral metastases. *J. Neurosurg.,* 8:411–422.
8. Antoni, N., and Lindgren, E. (1949): Steno's experiment in man as complication in lumbar aortography. *Acta Chir. Scand.,* 98:230–247.
9. Batson, O. V. (1940): The function of the vertebral veins and their rôle in the spread of metastases. *Ann. Surg.,* 112:138–149.
10. Batson, O. V. (1950): Discussion of paper by Guis & Grier. *Surgery,* 28:305–321.
11. Batson, O. V. (1957): The vertebral vein system. *Am. J. Roentgenol. Radium Ther. Nucl. Med.,* 78:195–212.

12. Billings, J., and Robertson, P. (1955): Paraplegia following chest surgery. *Aust. Ann. Med.*, 4:141–144.
13. Bolton, B. (1939): The blood supply of the human spinal cord. *J. Neurol. Psychiatry*, 2:137–148.
14. Brøbeck, O. (1950): Haemangioma of vertebra associated with compression of the spinal cord. *Acta Radiol. (Stockh)*, 34:235–243.
15. Boyarsky, S. (1954): Paraplegia following translumbar aortography. *JAMA*, 156:599–602.
16. Bucy, P. C., Heimburger, R. F., and Oberhill, H. R. (1948): Compression of the cervical spinal cord by herniated intervertebral discs. *J. Neurosurg.*, 5:471–492.
17. Chakravorty, B. G. (1969): Arterial supply to the cervical spinal cord and its relation to cervical myelopathy in spondylosis. *Ann. R. Coll. Surg. Engl.*, 45:232–251.
18. Chiurco, A. A. (1970): Multiple exostoses of bone with fatal spinal cord compression. *Neurology (Minneap)*, 20:275–278.
19. Clemens, H. J. (1961): *Die Venensysteme der menschlichen Wirbesäule.* de Gruyter, Berlin.
20. Craigie, E. H. (1938): The comparative anatomy and embryology of the capillary bed of the central nervous system. *Proc. Assoc. Res. Nerv. Ment. Dis.*, 18:1–28.
21. Crosby, E. C., Humphrey, T., and Lauer, E. W. (1962): *Correlative Anatomy of the Nervous System.* Macmillan, New York.
22. Denny-Brown, D., and Meyer, J. S. (1957): The cerebral collateral circulation. 2. Production of cerebral infarction by ischemic anoxia and its reversibility in early stages. *Neurology (Minneap)*, 7:567–579.
23. DiChiro, G., and Fried, L. C. (1971): Blood flow currents in spinal cord arteries. *Neurology (Minneap)*, 21:1088–1096.
24. Djørup, F. (1923): *Ganglieceller og Arterier. Cervikalpartiet af menneskets rygmorv.* Antal og Fordeling, Copenhagen.
25. Dodson, W. E., and Landau, W. M. (1973): Motor neuron loss due to aortic clamping in repair of coarctation. *Neurology (Minneap)*, 23:539–542.
26. Epstein, J. A., and Malis, L. I. (1955): Compression of spinal cord and cauda equina in achondroplastic dwarfs. *Neurology (Minneap)*, 5:875–881.
27. Evans, H. M. (1909): On the development of the aortae, cardinal and umbilical veins, and other blood vessels of vertebrate embryos from capillaries. *Anat. Rec.*, 3:498–518.
28. Fay, T. (1937): Epidural ascending spinal paralysis (Spiller's syndrome). *Trans. Am. Neurol. Assoc.*, 47–51.
29. Fried, L. C., and Aparicio, O. (1973): Experimental ischemia of spinal cord. *Neurology (Minneap)*, 23:289–293.
30. Gelfan, S., and Tarlov, I. M. (1955): Differential vulnerability of spinal cord structures to anoxia. *J. Neurophysiol.*, 18:170–188.
31. Gilles, F. H., and Nag, D. (1971): Vulnerability of human spinal cord in transient cardiac arrest. *Neurology (Minneap)*, 21:833–839.
32. Gillilan, L. A. (1958): The arterial blood supply of the human spinal cord. *J. Comp. Neurol.*, 110:75–103.
33. Gillilan, L. A. (1964): The correlation of the blood supply to the human brain stem with clinical brain stem lesions. *J. Neuropathol. Exp. Neurol.*, 23:78–108.
34. Gillilan, L. A. (1970): Veins of the spinal cord: Anatomic details; suggested clinical applications. *Neurology (Minneap)*, 20:860–868.
35. Gillilan, L. A. (1971): Arterial and venous anatomy of the spinal cord In: *Cerebral Vascular Diseases.* Grune & Stratton, New York.
36. Gillilan, L. A. (1976): Extra- and intra-cranial blood supply to brains of dog and cat. *Am. J. Anat.*, 146:237–254.
37. Greenfield, J. G., and Turner, J. W. A. (1939): Acute and subacute necrotic myelitis. *Brain*, 62:227–252.
38. Hallenbeck, J. M. (1976): Cinephotomicrography of dog spinal vessels during cord-damaging decompression sickness. *Neurology (Minneap)*, 26:191–199.
39. Hallenbeck, J. M., Bove, A. A., and Elliott, D. H. (1975): Mechanisms underlying spinal cord damage in decompression sickness. *Neurology (Minneap)*, 25:308–316.
40. Herren, R. Y., and Alexander, L. (1939): Sulcal and intrinsic blood vessels of human spinal cord. *Arch. Neurol. Psychiatry*, 41:678–687.

41. Heymans, C. (1955): Survival and revival of nervous tissues after arrest of circulation. *Physiol. Rev.,* 30:375–392.
42. His, W. (1887): Zur Geschichte des menschlichen Rückenmarkes und der Nervenwurzeln. *Abhandl. Math.-Phys. Cl. Sachs. Gesellsch. Wissensch.,* 13:477–514.
43. Hol, R., and Skjerven, O. (1954): Spinal cord damage in abdominal aortography. *Acta Radiol. (Stockh),* 42:276–284.
44. Hoskins, E. R. (1914): On the vascularization of the spinal cord of the pig. *Anat. Rec.,* 8:371–391.
45. Hughes, J. T. (1970): Thrombosis of the posterior spinal arteries. *Neurology (Minneap),* 20:659–664.
46. Hughes, J. T. (1971): Venous infarction of the spinal cord. *Neurology (Minneap),* 21:794–800.
47. Juba, A. (1938): Myelitis necroticans subacuta (Foix-Alajouanine). *Dtsch. Z. Nervenheilk.,* 148:17–30.
48. Kadyi, H. (1886): Über die Blutgefässe des menschlichen Rückenmarkes. *Anat. Anz.,* 1:304–314.
49. Kadyi, H. (1889): Über die Blutgefässe des menschlichen Rückenmarkes. In: *Nach einer im XV Bande der Denkschriften d. math.-naturw. Cl. d. Akad. d. Wissensch. in Krakau erschienenen Monographie, aus dem Polnischen Übersatzt vom Verfasser.* Gubrnowicz & Schmidt, Lemberg.
50. Kahn, E. A. (1947): The rôle of the dentate ligaments in spinal cord compression and the syndrome of lateral sclerosis. *J. Neurosurg.,* 4:191–199.
51. Katz, S. M., and Samuel, E. (1948): Varicosities of the spinal cord veins. *South Afr. Med. J.,* 22:507–509.
52. Kaufman, A. B., and Dunsmore, R. H. (1971): Clinicopathologic considerations in spinal meningeal calcification and ossification. *Neurology (Minneap),* 21:1243–1248.
53. Killen, D. A., and Foster, J. H. (1960): Spinal cord injury as a complication of aortography. *Ann. Surg.,* 152:211–230.
54. Kiloh, L. G. (1953): The syndromes of the arteries of the brain and spinal cord. Part II. *Postgrad. Med. J.,* 29:119–127.
55. Krogh, E. (1945): Studies on the blood supply to certain regions in the lumbar part of the spinal cord. *Acta Physiol. Scand.,* 10:271–281.
56. Krogh, E. (1950): The effect of acute hypoxia on the motor cells of the spinal cord. *Acta Physiol. Scand.,* 20:263–292.
57. Laufman, H., Berggren, R. E., Finley, T., and Anson, B. J. (1960): Anatomical studies of the lumbar arteries: With reference to the safety of translumbar aortography. *Ann. Surg.,* 152:621–634.
58. Lhermitte, J., Fribourg-Blanc, A., and Kyriaco, N. (1931): La gliose angéio-hypertrophique de la moelle épinière (myélite necrotique de Foix-Alajouanine). *Rev. Neurol. (Paris),* 2:37–53.
59. Mair, W. G. P., and Druckman, R. (1953): The pathology of spinal cord lesions and their relation to the clinical features in protrusion of cervical intervertebral discs. *Brain,* 76:70–91.
60. Mair, W. G. P., and Folkerts, J. F. (1953): Necrosis of the spinal cord due to thrombophlebitis (subacute necrotic myelitis). *Brain,* 76:563–575.
61. Nakanishi, T., Mannen, T., Toyokura, Y., Sakaguchi, R., and Tsuyama, N. (1974): Symptomatic ossification of the posterior longitudinal ligament of the cervical spine. *Neurology (Minneap),* 24:1139–1143.
62. Romanes, G. J. (1951): The motor cell columns of the lumbosacral spinal cord of the cat. *J. Comp. Neurol.,* 94:313–363.
63. Romanes, G. J. (1963): The arterial blood supply of the spinal cord, In: *Spinal Injuries,* edited by P. Harris. Proceedings of a symposium held in The Royal College of Surgeons of Edinburgh.
64. Russman, B. S., and Kazi, K. H. (1971): Spinal epidural hematoma and the Brown-Sequard syndrome. *Neurology (Minneap),* 21:1066–1068.
65. Sadka, M. (1953): Epidural spinal hemorrhage, with a report of two cases. *Med. J. Aust.,* 40:669–692.
66. Sahs, A. L. (1942): Vascular supply of the monkey's spinal cord. *J. Comp. Neurol.,* 76:403–415.

67. Schlapp, M. G. (1906): A case of ascending myelomalacia, caused by progressing venous thrombosis. *NY Med. J.*, 83:694–698.
68. Schlesinger, E. B., and Wood, E. H. (1952): Factors in the pathogenesis and diagnosis of spastic paraplegia due to cervical cord compression—the so-called "pseudo multiple sclerosis." *Trans. Am. Neurol. Assoc.*, 140–144.
69. Schneider, R. C. (1951): A syndrome in acute cervical spine injuries for which early operation is indicated. *J. Neurosurg.*, 8:360–367.
70. Schneider, R. C. (1955): The syndrome of acute anterior spinal injury. *J. Neurosurg.*, 12:95–122.
71. Spiller, W. G. (1911): Epidural ascending spinal paralysis. *Rev. Neurol. Psychiatry*, 9:494–498.
72. Steegmen, A. T. (1951): Clinical aspects of cerebral anoxia in man. *Neurology (Minneap)*, 1:261–274.
73. Steegmen, A. T. (1952): Syndrome of the anterior spinal artery. *Neurology (Minneap)*, 2:15–35.
74. Stern. W. E., and Rand, R. W. (1954): Spinal cord dysfunction from cervical intervertebral disk disease. *Neurology (Minneap)*, 4:883–893.
75. Suh, T. H., and Alexander, L. (1939): Vascular system of the human spinal cord. *Arch. Neurol. Psychiatry*, 41:659–677.
76. Tarlov, I. M., and Klinger, H. (1954): Spinal cord compression studies. II. Time limits for recovery after acute compression in dogs. *Arch. Neurol. Psychiatry*, 71:271–290.
77. Tureen, L. L. (1938): Circulation of the spinal cord and the effect of vascular occlusion. *Proc. Assoc. Res. Nerv. Ment. Dis.*, 18:394–437.
78. Van Gehuchten, P. (1927): Un cas de myélite nécrotique aiguë (étude clinique et anatomo-pathologique). *Rev. Neurol. (Paris)*, 1:505–519.
79. Verbiest, H. (1954): A radicular syndrome from developmental narrowing of the lumbar vertebral canal. *J. Bone Joint Surg.*, 36-B:230–237.
80. Woodard, J. S., and Freeman, L. W. (1956): Ischemia of the spinal cord: An experimental study. *J. Neurosurg.*, 13:63–72.
81. Woolam, D. H. M., and Millen, J. W. (1955): The arterial supply of the spinal cord and its significance. *J. Neurol. Neurosurg. Psychiatry*, 18:97–102.
82. Yoss, R. E. (1950): Vascular supply of the spinal cord: The production of vascular syndromes. *U. Mich. Med. Bull.*, 16:333–345.

Spinal Deformities and Neurological Dysfunction, edited by S. N. Chou and E. L. Seljeskog. Raven Press, New York © 1978.

Spinal Mechanics (Flexibility and Stability)

James M. Morris

Department of Orthopaedic Surgery, University of California San Francisco, San Francisco, California 94143

The vertebral column is a remarkable structure. Although normally quite flexible, it can be rigid and capable of withstanding great forces. Consider, for example, the function of the vertebral column in the wrestler compared with that in the weight lifter.

In an engineering sense the spinal column possesses a number of unique features. First, it is not a homogeneous structure, but instead is composed of relatively rigid units (vertebrae) interspaced with highly deformable discs arranged within a complex of guiding and restraining facet joints. This combination of strength and flexibility is a workable compromise that affords maximal protection for the spinal cord and nerve with minimal restriction of mobility. Second, the spine is not straight but rather is curved to adapt to our upright posture. This feature allows the column to damp vertical shocks (e.g., those imposed by running or jumping) more efficiently. If the spine were straight, these shocks would be transmitted along the axis of the spine and truly be a jolting experience for the head. The curvature of the column allows it to bend as well as compress. The third major feature of the spine is the variation in its size and geometry. The spine is not only tapered, but the very geometry of vertebrae and facets places definite restrictions on the possible motions between segments.

The spinal column serves as a sustaining rod for the maintenance of the upright position of the body and, as such, is subject to many forces of different types (e.g., compression, tension, shear, bending, and rotation). It is provided with (a) an intrinsic stability by the interplay of disc and ligament forces, and (b) an extrinsic stability by the trunk musculature, especially that of the abdomen and thoracic cage.

GROSS ANATOMY OF THE SPINE

The bones of the spinal column consist of 24 presacral vertebrae, the sacrum, and the coccyx. The presacral segments increase in size from the first cervical to the 5th lumbar vertebra, whereas sacral and coccygeus segments decrease in size from the first sacral segment caudally. A typical

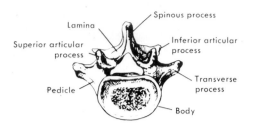

Lamina
Spinous process
Superior articular process
Inferior articular process
Transverse process
Pedicle
Body

FIG. 1. Fifth lumbar vertebra. (From ref. 7.)

presacral vertebra is composed of four parts (Fig. 1): (a) the body, which is primarily for transmission of forces; (b) the laminae and pedicles, which with the body enclose the spinal canal; (c) the spinous and transverse processes, for attachment of muscles and ligaments; and (d) the posterior articular processes, or posterior articular facets, which guide and limit motion between adjacent vertebrae. The adult spine typically demonstrates four curves in the sagittal plane: cervical lordosis, thoracic kyphosis, lumbar lordosis, and sacral kyphosis.

The vertebrae articulate by means of a complex joint which includes: (a) the intervertebral disc anteriorly, and (b) the two posterior articulations between the facets, which are of the gliding type and which possess true synovial joint cavities. The articular facets of the vertebra above generally overlie the superior facets of the vertebra below.

A series of ligaments placed under tension by expanding intradiscal pressure firmly bind the vertebral segments together. These ligaments include: (a) a longitudinal system that binds all vertebrae together into a mechanical unit, i.e., the anterior and posterior longitudinal ligaments and the supraspinous ligament; and (b) a longitudinal system that secures one segment to another, i.e., the interspinal, intertransverse, and iliolumbar ligaments and the ligamentum flavum. This two-system arrangement accounts for the relative stability of the spine when devoid of musculature.

STRUCTURE AND COMPOSITION
OF THE INTERVERTEBRAL DISC

The intervertebral disc, which gives the spine its flexibility, is generally considered to consist of three components: the nucleus pulposus, which occupies the central 50 to 60% of the cross-sectional area of the disc; the surrounding, thick anulus fibrosus; and the two cartilaginous end-plates, which separate the disc from the vertebral bodies above and below it. Many authors consider the end-plates to be a portion of the vertebral body rather than of the disc. There is no doubt, however, that the integrity of the nucleus depends on the integrity of the end-plates.

Located in the posterior central portion of the disc, the nucleus pulposus is an oval gelatinous mass consisting of chondrocyte-like cell bodies dispersed within an intercellular matrix made up of poorly differentiated collagen fibrils that are surrounded by a protein polysaccharide complex. The polysaccharide is generally chondroitin sulfate. Because of its polar (–OH) groups, the nucleus has a great capacity to imbibe and bind water (depending on its age, the nucleus pulposus contains 69–88% water by weight).

The anulus fibrosus is formed of successive layers of collagenous and fibrocartilaginous tissue which are firmly anchored to the vertebrae above and below. The fibers within the layers are directed obliquely between the vertebrae, and successive layers of fibers are perpendicular to those of the adjacent layer, an orientation that gives the disc its elasticity. The layers of fibrous tissue are normally firmly bound together by an intercellular cement-like substance. The anterior and lateral portions of the anulus are approximately twice as thick as the posterior portion, where the layers are fewer in number and the fibers are oriented in a direction more nearly parallel to those of the adjacent level. There is also less binding substance in the posterior portion. These conditions no doubt contribute to the propensity of the disc to herniate posteriorly. Fibers of the innermost layers in the anulus pass into the nucleus and blend with the intercellular matrix, resulting in a lack of demarcation of the anulus and nucleus.

BIOMECHANICS OF THE INTERVERTEBRAL JOINT

The intervertebral joint complex has six possible degrees of freedom, three in rotation and three in translation. Because of the anatomic configuration of the joint complex, certain motions occur more easily than others. Compression, lateral bending, anterior/posterior bending, and torsion occur most readily, whereas tension and anterior/posterior and lateral shear are more restricted in the normal joint (5). Experimental studies on cadaver spines demonstrated that the posterior facets play a relatively minor role in withstanding pure compressive force (3). The intervertebral disc is the structure responsible for transmission of the compressive forces. It is well suited for this task since it is capable of sustaining enormous forces without loss of mechanical function. It is so strong that laboratory tests on cadaver discs have failed to crush them irreversibly before failure of the vertebral bodies. During compression-loading studies of a disc and adjacent vertebral bodies *in vitro,* the first structure to fail is the end-plate, usually by one or more cracks that allow escape of nuclear material into the spongiosa. Failure occurs at compressive loads of 453.6 to 635.0 kg (1,000 to 1,400 lb) in healthy lumbar discs from young persons and at lower loads in specimens demonstrating disc degeneration or osteoporosis. As the compression forces increase, the next structure to fail is the vertebral body itself, with compression of spicules of the spongiosa or complete loss of structural integrity. The amount of the force ranges from 589.7 to 1,088.6 kg (1,000 to 2,400 lb) for healthy lumbar specimens. The significant factor here is that in a normal disc irreparable damage cannot be produced by compression alone; no intact intervertebral disc specimen has been experimentally herniated.

VISCOELASTICITY

In addition to the study of the failure load of the disc-vertebral complex, the response of the disc to lower loads is important. The disc and, to a lesser extent, the vertebral body demonstrate viscoelastic properties characteristic of biological materials in general. This property is probably best demonstrated by the *load-deflection* curve for pure compression (Fig. 2). When a compression load is plotted against deflection or deformation of the disc, the curve does not show the steady increase in deflection proportionate to the increasing force that would be indicated by a straight line. It demonstrates, however, stiffening behavior, the stiffness being the slope or rate of increase of load, with deformation measured in units of kilograms per millimeter (pounds per inch). The tangent or slope of the curve increases as the curve bends upward, indicating stiffening of the disc as a result of loading. Most engineering materials have a curve that tends to flatten or "soften" for high loads; thus the disc is unique as a compressive unit.

Another important feature of the load-deflection curve is its dependence on loading rate. The disc becomes stiffer the faster it is loaded. This impor-

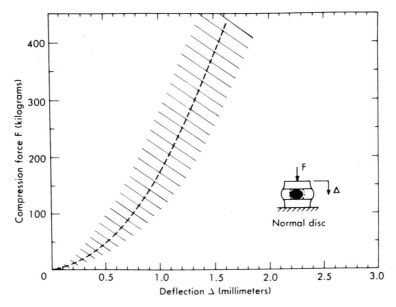

FIG. 2. An average force-deflection curve for compression of 24 normal discs. Range of variation is indicated by the shaded area. (From ref. 8.)

tant feature appears to have value in such an instance as high-speed ejection from a jet aircraft.

The disc exhibits other phenomena characteristic of viscoelasticity: *creep* and *load relaxation*. Creep refers to the tendency to compress with time under constant compressive loading. This long-term compressive deformation of the disc is responsible for the change in height of an individual between morning and evening. This creep behavior is probably due to fluid transfer into and out of the disc as a result of the hydrophilic nature of the nucleus. Load relaxation refers to the decrease of load as a function of time for a constant deformation.

The contributions to spinal mechanics of the components of the intervertebral disc (i.e., the nucleus and the anulus) have been studied with interesting results (6). It has been visually observed that the first time the disc is compressed in a load-deflection test after a small defect has been made in the anulus, nuclear material is extruded through the opening. The deflection curve is noted to be much softer, indicating that the disc is more compressible than normal for a given load. If the load is removed and the disc is then loaded in the same manner, the disc becomes stiffer; by the third loading cycle, normal compressive behavior is restored. However, because of loss of nuclear material, the disc is now slightly diminished in height despite a normal load-deflection curve. Similar findings were observed if the nucleus pulposus was removed, as would be done in a laminotomy or discectomy.

Of particular interest in this study was the behavior of the anulus after

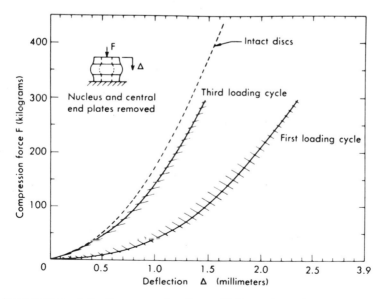

FIG. 3. Average force-deflection curves for discs with the anulus only remaining, repeated loading. Ranges of variation are indicated by the shaded areas. (From ref. 6.)

removal of the nucleus, the end-plates, and the supporting bone above and below the end-plates (Fig. 3). This preparation excluded any possibility of a self-contained generation of pressure within the nucleus. Again, the first time the disc was compressed a very soft curve was revealed, indicating that the anulus was compressed into a new configuration. For the third loading cycle, the load-deflection curve approached that of a normal disc. These results indicate that the anulus alone is strong enough to carry the compressive force on the disc in a normal fashion. The role of the nucleus therefore appears to be one of load distribution rather than direct load-carrying. In addition, the imbibition pressure of the nucleus serves to maintain the height of a normal disc and preserves normal ligament tension and facet alignment. This study helps to explain how most patients, at least initially, are able to do so well after discectomy. Note, however, that this is an *in vivo* study, and the effects of rotation and shear have not been determined.

BENDING

Bending (i.e., flexion, extension, lateral bending) is the second most common motion of the intervertebral joint complex. The mechanics of these motions may be characterized by a curve similar to that of force versus deflection for axial compression. In bending movements the motion observed is rotation, measured in degrees, and the force acting to produce this rotation is called moment. A moment is a force applied in such a way as to produce rotation about a fixed point: the value of the moment (given in units of newton-meters or foot-pounds) is force × distance of the lever arm. A curve of a moment-rotation test is similar to that of a force-deflection test. The rotation response of an *in vitro* intervertebral joint demonstrates behavior characteristic of collagenous biological materials. The curves are nonlinear, with increasing stiffness, as noted for the force-deflection curves. The importance of the posterior facets for bending varies with the particular motion. For lateral bending and flexion, the curves vary slightly but are essentially the same. The facets, however, have a definite stiffening influence on extension in both the lumbar and thoracic regions (approximately three times that for a joint with the facets removed). This stiffening effect appears to be attributable to facet joint compression and impingement as the joint is extended with resulting resistance to further rotation.

TORSION

Torsion, or rotation, of the intervertebral joint about its long axis is a complex motion dependent on the structural features of the posterior facets. Torsion in the thoracic and lumbar joints differs significantly because of differences in the facet orientation (Fig. 4). In the thoracic spine the center of rotation lies within the nucleus, and the disc is subjected to rotation forces.

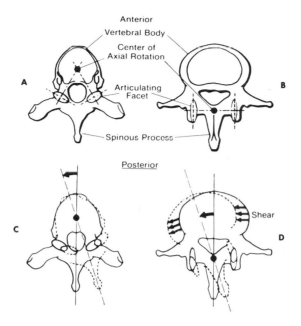

FIG. 4. Mechanism of axial rotation (**C** and **D**) in thoracic (*left*) and a lumbar (*right*) vertebra. (From ref. 2.)

In the lumbar spine the center of axial rotation lies posterior to the disc, and the disc is thus subject to translational shearing forces. In the case of bending, stiffening characterizes the response to a moment. The torsional behavior of the thoracic and lumbar discs was tested before and after removal of posterior facets (Fig. 5). The thoracic joint showed little change in

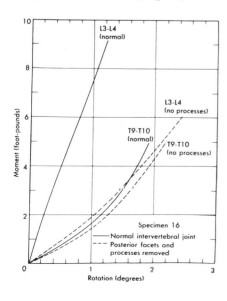

FIG. 5. Effect of articular processes and posterior elements on moment-rotation behavior of a thoracic and a lumbar intervertebral joint in torsion. (1 foot-pound = 0.138 kg-meter.) (From ref. 5.)

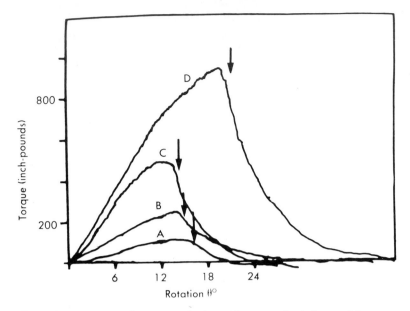

FIG. 6. Typical moment-rotation curves for intact intervertebral disc and its components loaded to failure. **A,** intact joints between articular processes with capsule of contralateral articular process removed. **B,** ruptured isolated disc. **C,** intact (normal) isolated disc. **D,** intact intervertebral joint with a normal discogram. (1 inch-pound = 0.0115 kg-meter.) (From ref. 1.)

torsional (moment rotation) behavior as a result of facet removal. This was to be expected since the facet articulating surfaces of the thoracic facets are horizontal in orientation and thus offer little resistance to torsion. The lumbar facets, however, are aligned in the sagittal plane and resist torsional or rotational motions. Torsional tests by Farfan indicate an average failure torque of 881×10^6 dyne-cm, or 8.99 kg/meter. He estimates that the disc provides 40 to 50% of the torsional stiffness, with the remainder provided by the posterior facet joints. When torsion was applied to the point of failure (Fig. 6), it was found that intervertebral joints with degenerated discs were, as expected, weaker than normal specimens.

AXIAL ROTATION OF THE SPINE IN VIVO

Gregersen and Lucas (2) studied axial rotation of the spine *in vivo* while the trunk was rotated from side to side. Steinmann pins were inserted in the spinous processes under local anesthesia, and angular displacement between various vertebral segments was measured by special transducers designed to measure only rotation. Approximately 74° of rotation occurred between the 1st and 12th thoracic vertebrae, and the average cumulative rotation from the sacrum to the first thoracic vertebra was 102° (Fig. 7).

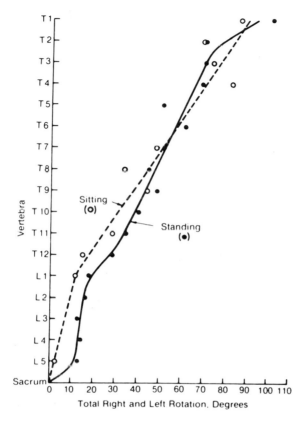

FIG. 7. Maximum total axial rotation of thoracolumbar spine in standing and sitting positions, pelvis immobilized. (From ref. 2.)

Very little rotation occurs in the lumbar as compared with the thoracic spine, and again this is a reflection of the orientation of the facet joints. Similar measurements obtained during walking indicated the following: (a) The pelvis and the lumbar spine rotate as a functional unit. (b) In the lower thoracic spine, rotation diminishes gradually up to the 7th thoracic vertebra. (c) The 7th thoracic vertebra represents the area of transition from vertebral rotation in the direction of the pelvis to rotation in the opposite direction— that of the shoulder girdle (Fig. 8). (d) The amount of rotation in the upper thoracic spine increases gradually from the 7th to the 1st thoracic vertebra.

Using a specially designed transducer, Lumsden and Morris (4) measured axial rotation at the lumbosacral level *in vivo*. Approximately 6° of rotation occurred at the lumbosacral joint during maximal rotation. With the pelvis fixed, the subject stood or else straddled a bicycle seat. Approximately 1.5° of rotation occurred during normal walking. Rotation at the lumbosacral joint was not measurably affected by asymmetrically oriented lumbar facets

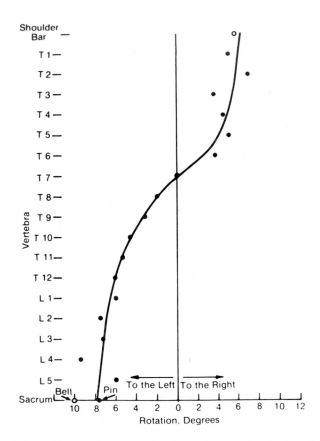

FIG. 8. Axial rotation of thoracolumbar spine during locomotion. Left heel strike to right heel strike, 4.38 km/hr. Solid circles = Values for readings from pins. Open circles = Readings from belt. (From ref. 2.)

(tropism). It was always associated with flexion of the 5th lumbar vertebra on the sacrum.

THE LIGAMENTOUS SPINE

The isolated spinal column, devoid of musculature, demonstrates an intrinsic stability. This stability is provided by the opposing forces of the intradiscal pressure (due to imbibition) and the tension within the ligaments of the spinal column.

The ligamentous spine behaves as a modified elastic rod. Although the spinal column is nonuniform in size, bending and compression stiffnesses are nearly constant throughout the dorsolumbar spine. This results from the

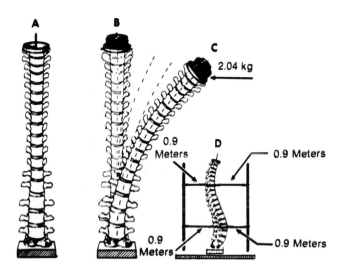

FIG. 9. Adult thoracolumbar ligamentous spine, fixed at base and free at top, under vertical loading, and restrained at midthoracic and midlumbar levels in anteroposterior plane. **A,** before loading. **B,** during loading. **C,** stability failure occurring under 2.04-kg load. **D,** lateral view showing anteroposterior restraints. (Courtesy of D. B. Lucas and B. Bresler.)

fact that the elasticity of the disc is roughly proportional to the height of the disc and inversely proportional to the cross-sectional area of the disc. If both the height and the cross-sectional areas increase from T1 to L5, the result is a constancy in bending and compressive stiffness, an unusual feature in a tapered column.

Torsional stiffness, however, is not uniform; as a result of the orientation of their facets, the lower lumbar joints are far stiffer than the thoracic joints. The upper thoracic vertebrae (T10 and above) articulate with the rib cage in such a manner that resistance to torsional motion is increased. The thoracic vertebrae may be visualized as a rigid unit bound together by the rib cage. Since the lumbar vertebrae possess an inherently high torsional stiffness, they may also be considered as a stiff structural unit. This leaves the discs in the 10th to the 12th thoracic vertebrae as the intermediate elastic elements when sudden torsional moments are applied, such as might occur within the column during a fall or during acceleration. These intermediate discs are likely to absorb a great deal of energy since rotation is greatest at these levels. Thus the lowest thoracic discs are the most prone to injuries involving torsion.

As mentioned, the ligamentous spine possesses an intrinsic stability. This stability, however, is minimal so far as the entire column is concerned, for although the ligamentous spine is capable of standing erect without external support, a compressive force of only 2.0 kg (4.5 lb) applied to the top is enough to buckle the column laterally (Fig. 9).

ROLE OF THE TRUNK IN SPINE STABILITY

If the ligamentous spine is able to withstand only very small loads, it is apparent that the extrinsic support provided by the trunk musculature is responsible for the ability of the spinal column to withstand the great loads to which it may be exposed.

When an individual bends forward to lift a heavy weight, a large force is generated at the lumbosacral junction. This force results largely from the contraction of the erector spinae musculature acting through a very short lever arm. A static free-body diagram can be used to calculate the amount of force at the lumbosacral level. For example, if a weight of 90.7 kg (200 lb) is lifted, assuming that the ratio of the anterior to the posterior lever arm is approximately 10:1, there is (theoretically at least) a force of approximately 907.2 kg (2,000 lb) at the lumbosacral level (the values in Fig. 10 are slightly higher). However, a number of biomechanical experiments have been carried out to determine the strength of the discs and vertebral bodies, and it has been demonstrated that such great forces cannot be tolerated. By placing two vertebral bodies and their intervening disc in a materials-testing compression machine or subjecting them suddenly to dynamic forces, considerable information has been obtained.

Compression forces have been imposed up to the point of failure of a particular section of the spine being studied. This failure is characterized by an audible crack followed by sanguineous leakage from one of the vertebrae (usually the superior) through the vascular foramen and occasionally at some

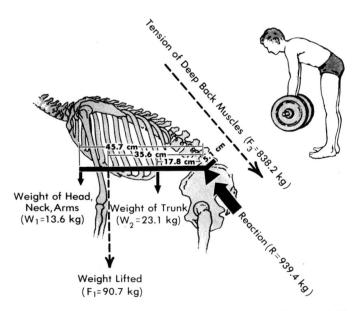

FIG. 10. Force on lower lumbar part of spine, with role of trunk omitted. (From ref. 9.)

point along the attachment of the peripheral fibers of the anulus to the vertebral body. The evidence of failure is often difficult to visualize either during gross examination or roentgenographically. It may consist of compression of a few spicules of bone, cracks in the end-plate, or sometimes collapse of the plate. It has been shown that failure occurs in specimens from young persons at a compressive load of 453.6 to 771.1 kg (1,000 to 1,700 lb). When specimens from older persons were studied, the critical load was found to be much less, even as little as 136.1 kg (300 lb). However, it is important to note that when the anulus is intact its elastic limits cannot be exceeded without vertebral fracture. Because the end-plate is the component most susceptible to fracture as a result of the forces exerted on the spine, this structure generally gives way first. It is most likely to fracture centrally when the disc is normal and when the resistance of the vertebral body is greater than the pressure generated within the nucleus. This type of end-plate failure might explain the origin of Schmorl's nodules in young people. Peripheral plate fractures or fissures across the end-plate occur when various degrees of disc degeneration that are present lead to an abnormal distribution of forces across the disc space.

The vertebral body itself is the next most susceptible part of the segment under study and usually collapses before herniation of the nucleus occurs through the anulus. Even when well-developed defects of the anulus are present, end-plate or vertebral fractures are more likely to occur than disc herniation (note that the above values are not *in vivo* measurements). It has also been shown experimentally in dogs that a single violent trauma causes fracture of the vertebra more often than disc herniation. This agrees well with the opinion that trauma per se seldom causes disc herniation. Organic as well as inorganic materials generally are able to withstand stresses during a short period more readily than stresses exerted over a longer period. It has been demonstrated that an approximately equal number of end-plate fractures occurred when a static force of approximately 589.7 kg (1,300 lb) was exerted as when dynamic stresses of 1,179.3 kg (2,600 lb) were applied. This similarity of result is no doubt related to the viscoelastic properties of the structures involved.

How then can the spine support the theoretical loads to which it may be subjected? One explanation for the ability of the spine to withstand such forces is to consider it as a segmented elastic column supported by the paraspinal muscles and situated within and attached to the sides of two chambers, the abdominal and thoracic cavities, which are separated by the diaphragm. The abdominal cavity is filled with a combination of solids and liquids, whereas the thoracic cavity is filled largely with fluids and air. The action of the trunk musculature converts these chambers into semirigid walled cylinders of air and semisolids capable of transmitting forces generated in loading the spine and thereby relieving the spinal column itself.

This hypothesis was studied utilizing small balloon-tip catheters to

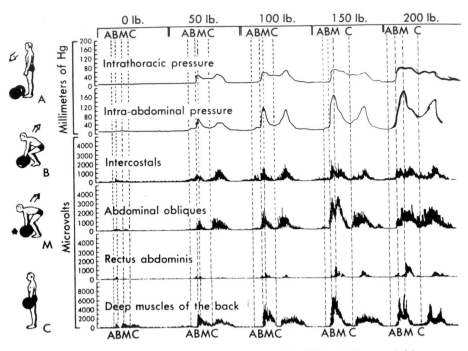

FIG. 11. Dynamic loading of spine. (1 pound = 0.45 kg.) (From ref. 9.)

measure the intrathoracic (esophageal) and intraabdominal (stomach) pressures (9). It was possible to show that during the act of lifting the action of intercostal muscles and muscles of the shoulder girdle rendered the thoracic cage quite rigid. An increase in thoracic pressure resulted, converting the thoracic cage and the spine into a sturdy unit capable of transmitting large forces. The abdominal contents were compressed into a semirigid mass by contraction of the diaphragm and muscles of the abdominal wall, thereby making the abdominal cavity a semirigid cylinder. The force of the weights lifted by the arms is thus transmitted to the spinal column by the muscles of the shoulder girdle, principally by the trapezius, and then to the abdominal cylinder and the pelvis, partly through the spinal column and partly through the rigid rib cage and abdomen. The larger the weight lifted, or the greater the static loading of the spine (pulling on a strain ring), the greater was the activity of the trunk musculature. There was also a concomitant increase in the intracavitary pressures (Fig. 11). With regard to the effects of the increased cavitary pressures, the calculated force on the lumbosacral disc during the lifting of a heavy load was decreased by 30% and the load on the lower thoracic spine was approximately 50% less than it would have been without the support by the trunk. Thus when 90.7 kg (200 lb) is lifted, only 640.4 kg (1,408 lb) of force is actually transmitted along the spine to the lumbosacral level, instead of the theoretical force of

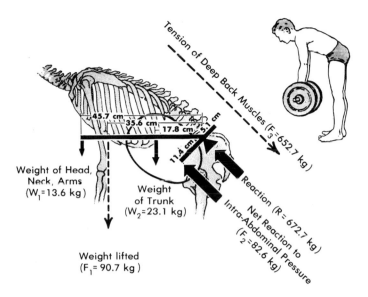

FIG. 12. Force on lower lumbar part of spine, with role of trunk included. (From ref. 9.)

approximately 907.2 kg (2,000 lb) (Fig. 12). It is interesting to note that when a tight corset is worn about the abdomen an increase in the intra-abdominal and intrathoracic pressures resulted from tightening of the corset. At the same time, during the act of lifting there was a decrease in activity of the thoracic and abdominal muscles, indicating that the effect of the muscle can be replaced by such an external appliance.

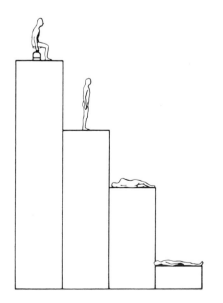

FIG. 13. Approximate relationship between position and total pressure on normal third and fourth lumbar discs. Positions shown are sitting, standing, reclining (with tilting), and lying with complete muscle relaxation (in one subject under general anesthesia, with the use of additional muscle relaxants, the pressure recorded was similar to that obtained from autopsy specimens). (From ref. 11.)

In an attempt to confirm the above calculations, intradiscal pressures were measured *in vivo* by Nachemson and Morris (11). A needle with a pressure-sensitive polyethylene membrane tip was inserted into the disc under study. Intradiscal pressure of 10 to 15 kg/cm² was found in normal discs with subjects in a sitting position. There was approximately 30% less pressure during standing, and 50% less in a reclining position (Fig. 13). From the measurements one can determine that the lower lumbar discs of adults must support total loads of as much as 99.8–174.6 kg (220–385 lb) when the subjects are seated. For the standing position, total loads of 90.7–120.2 kg (200–265 lb) were calculated from the pressure values obtained. The intradiscal pressure was significantly elevated when weights were lifted and especially when lifting involved forward flexion of the trunk. The figures obtained agree closely with the theoretical calculations of forces on the spine mentioned previously. Nachemson and Elfström (10) recently extended this study to record intradiscal pressures during a variety of tasks or activities.

REFERENCES

1. Farfan, H. F., Cosette, J. W., Robertson, G. H., Wells, R. V., and Kraus, H. (1970): The effects of torsion on the lumbar intervertebral joints: The role of torsion in the production of disc degeneration. *J. Bone Joint Surg.*, 52A:468–497.
2. Gregersen, G. G., and Lucas, D. B. (1967): An *in vivo* study of the axial rotation of the human thoracolumbar spine. *J. Bone Joint Surg.*, 49A:247–262.
3. Hirsch, C., and Nachemson, A. (1954): New observations on the mechanical behavior of lumbar discs. *Acta Orthop. Scand.*, 23:254–283.
4. Lumsden, R. M., II, and Morris, J. M. (1968): An *in vivo* study of axial rotation and immobilization at the lumbosacral joint. *J. Bone Joint Surg.*, 50A:1591–1602.
5. Markolf, K. L. (1972): Deformation of the thoracolumbar intervertebral joints in response to external loads: A biomechanical study using autopsy material. *J. Bone Joint Surg.*, 54A:511–533.
6. Markolf, K. L., and Morris, J. M. (1974): The structural components of the intervertebral disc: A study of their contributions to the ability of the disc to withstand compressive forces. *J. Bone Joint Surg.*, 56A:675–687.
7. Morris, J. M. (1973): Biomechanics of the spine. *Arch. Surg.*, 107:418–423.
8. Morris, J. M., and Markolf, K. L. (1975): Biomechanics of the lumbosacral spine. In: *Atlas of Orthotics: Biomechanical Principles and Application*, pp. 312–331. Mosby, St. Louis.
9. Morris, J. M., Lucas, D. B., and Bresler, B. (1961): Role of the trunk in stability of the spine. *J. Bone Joint Surg.*, 43A:327–351.
10. Nachemson, A., and Elfström, G. (1970): Intravital dynamic pressure measurements in lumbar discs: A study of common movements, maneuvers and exercises. *Scand. J. Rehabil. Med. (Suppl. 1)*, 1:1–40.
11. Nachemson, A., and Morris, J. M. (1964): *In vivo* measurements of intradiscal pressure: Discometry, a method for the determination of pressure in the lower lumbar discs. *J. Bone Joint Surg.*, 46A:1077–1092.

Spinal Deformities and Neurological
Dysfunction, edited by S. N. Chou and E. L.
Seljeskog. Raven Press, New York © 1978.

Developmental Abnormalities
of Spinal Cord and Vertebral Column

John E. Lonstein

*Department of Orthopaedic Surgery, University of Minnesota, Minneapolis,
Minnesota 55455 and Twin Cities Scoliosis Center,
Minneapolis, Minnesota 55454*

Normally the vertebra are placed one on top of the other without lateral curvature. *Scoliosis* refers to a curvature of the spinal column in the upright position, and *kyphosis* to a posterior angulation of the vertebral column. This is normal to a certain degree in the thoracic area and may be increased, but any increase in the cervical or lumbar area is definitely abnormal. *Lordosis* is an anterior angulation of the vertebral column and occurs normally in the cervical and lumbar areas. It may be increased in these areas, or it may occur in the thoracic area, any degree of which here being abnormal. Numerous diseases are associated with spinal deformities. A spinal deformity is regarded as a symptom of an underlying lesion and does not constitute a diagnosis itself.

Table 1 gives a partial list of the etiology of scoliosis, kyphosis, and lordosis. The commonest etiology of scoliosis is idiopathic, comprising approximately 80% of cases. Congenital and neuromuscular types are the next most common. A full description of these abnormalities is impossible here, so attention is turned to two groups that are of importance to orthopedic surgeons and neurosurgeons: the developmental anomalies of spinal cord and vertebral column, and the postlaminectomy spine deformities.

INTRODUCTION

From the description of the embryology of the spinal cord and vertebral column, it is seen that dynamic changes occur simultaneously in various parts of the embryo within a short period of time. Stages in vertebral column and spinal cord growth are related owing to inductive influences. The notochord induces formation of the vertebral bodies from the sclerotome cells that migrate from the somite. The neural tube induces formation of the posterior arch from the surrounding mesoderm. If the notochord is excised experimentally there is abnormal development of the vertebral bodies, resulting in a continuous nonsegmented bony sheet without differentiation.

41

TABLE 1. *Classification of spine deformities*

Scoliosis
  Idiopathic
  Neuromuscular
    Neuropathic
    Myopathic
  Congenital
  Neurofibromatosis
  Mesenchymal
  Traumatic
  Soft tissue contracture
  Osteochondrystrophies
  Tumor
  Metabolic
  Lumbosacral abnormality
  Thoracogenic
  Hysterical
  Postural
Kyphosis
  Postural
  Scheuermann's disease
  Congenital
  Paralytic
  Posttraumatic
  Infection
  Postlaminectomy
  Metabolic
  Tumor
Lordosis
  Postural
  Postlaminectomy
  Contractures
  Congenital

Posterior arches form normally around the neural tube. Ablation of the neural tube affects the appearance of these arches. The vertebral bodies form normally, without formation of vertebral arches posteriorly.

SPINAL CORD ABNORMALITIES

Spinal cord abnormalities (4,11) that occur during the stage of neurulation result in nervous tissue being external on the embryo without skin coverage. Abnormalities that occur during later stages of canalization or retrogressive differentiation have an intact skin coverage. The three important lesions most commonly seen are myelodysplasia, diastematomyelia, and the spinal dysraphism group.

Myelodysplasia

Myelodysplasia falls in the group of open neural tube lesions. Theories regarding its development fall into two categories: (a) that the neural tube never undergoes normal closure, remaining open completely or partially; and (b) that the neural tube closes normally and some mechanism occurs with reopening of the neural tube.

A majority of neuroembryologists postulate that the neural tube never closes (10,11,14). Specimens from spontaneous and therapeutic abortions in humans provide evidence to support this theory. Embryos have been recovered which on examination show an open neural tube at a stage when the neural tube should have closed. These findings were in very early embryos, and it appeared that the folding and closure process had not taken place in this area. In addition, Patten (14) observed an overgrowth of nervous tissue in some cases of open lesions, providing an explanation of why the neural tubes did not fuse properly. There is an overgrowth of neuroectoderm over the surface ectoderm at the edge of the open lesion. The question is whether this overgrowth is primary (i.e., preventing normal closure) or secondary (i.e., occurring after failure of closure).

Gardner (5,6) proposed that normal neurulation is followed by an abnormal process in which opening or rupture occurs. He believes that the thin roof of the fourth ventricle of the brain becomes impermeable to the passage of cerebrospinal fluid (CSF), with resulting accumulation. This results in increased pressure in the central canal of the spinal cord (hydroencephalomyelia). With this distention and abnormal pressure, the covering of the neural tube ruptures, resulting in formation of myelodysplasia.

Padget (12,13) recently theorized that the neural tube closes normally, and then a cleft appears in the dorsal neural tube allowing escape of CSF in the subectodermal space. This ectoderm could secondarily rupture, with exposure of the neural tube to the amniotic cavity. Padget termed this process "neuroschisis."

The lesions seen in this group with abnormalities in the process of neurulation present with an open neural tube without intact skin coverage. These lesions include craniorachis, which is the most severe, with failure of closure of the whole neural tube. This abnormality is incompatible with further embryological development. Cranially the lesion seen with failure of closure of the anterior neuropore is anencephaly.

In the area of the posterior neuropore, there is an open neural plate with an overgrowth of neural tissue. A large number of patients have in addition an Arnold-Chiari malformation involving the cerebellum and medulla at the foramen magnum. The varieties of meningomyelocele can be differentiated depending on the level of the lesion and the extent of the open defect. It must be noted that, although normal ectoderm is absent over the sac, the surrounding epithelium does proliferate, covering these lesions from the periphery to the center. Epithelialization can thus occur, but no skin integuments are present that would be derived from the normal mesoderm. These lesions include the myelocele, meningocele, and the myelomeningocele. The differentiation depends on the extent to which the spinal cord is involved in the lesion.

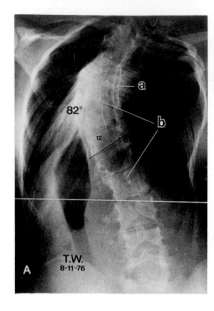

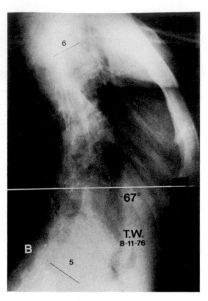

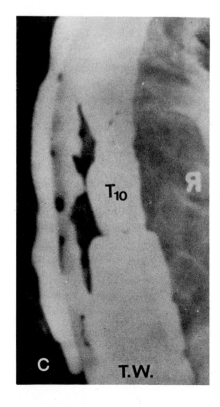

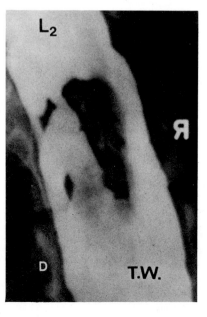

Diastematomyelia

Diastematomyelia (1,2,9) refers to lesions in which the spinal cord is split in some portion. The area of division can be over a long or a short portion of the spinal cord. James and Lassman (9) divided these lesions into two types: (a) where each cord was invested with a separate dura mater; and (b) where both cords were in one dural tube. In most cases with separate dural tubes, a bony, cartilagenous, or fibrous septum was present occupying the space between the two dural sacs (Fig. 1). When there was a single dural tube, no septum was present. In this group there were anomalous bands of dense fibrous tissue or abnormal dorsal nerve roots. These bands were usually located between the spinal cord and the neural arch.

The etiology of this lesion was proposed by Bremer (1) and Cohen and Sledge (2) to be persistence of the neurenteric canal. This canal exists at the stage of formation of the initial notochord when breakdown of the ventral cells of the notochord allow communication between the yolk sac and the amniotic cavity. If a portion of this connection remains, the spinal cord and vertebral centrum develop on either side of this connection. The vertebral centra on either side develop normally and attempt to form separate completed vertebral bodies. In the midline the two vertebrae attempt to form pedicles, and these fuse forming a fibrous, cartilagenous, or bony septum that lies in the split of the neural tube. This can be only a spur on the posterior surface of the vertebral body, or it may extend to the ectoderm, connecting the ectoderm to the posterior surface of the vertebral body; the latter usually is a fibrous band. It is common for skin changes to occur overlying this abnormality (see below).

Gardner (7,8) implicates nonpermeability of the fourth ventricular roof with hydrocephalomyelia as the cause of diastematomyelia. This distention of the central canal results in rupture of the distal neural tube, forming two separate spinal cords and a diastematomyelia. This theory is not widely accepted.

The role of the notochord in the development of this split neural tube is unknown. Experimentally it has been shown that excision of Hensen's node (from which the notochord develops) is associated with duplication of the neural tube. Completely separate spinal cords, notochords, and vertebrae form. Associated with the split neural tube is tethering of the spinal cord by

---

FIG. 1. T. W. A diastematomyelia and failure of segmentation. **A:** Anteroposterior x-ray showing a large unsegmented bar on the right (a) with a 82° left thoracic curve. Note that the spinal canal is widened in the thoracic area and upper lumbar area with obvious bony spurs (b). **B:** Lateral standing x-ray shows thoracic lordosis. The combination of scoliosis and lordosis is due to the fact that the area of failure of segmentation is posterolateral, involving the pedicles, laminae, and apophyseal joints on one side. **C** and **D.** Myelogram shows the filling defects seen with two at the lower thoracic and one in the upper lumbar spine.

the cartilage, bone, or fibrous tissue at the distal end of the split, which can result in a neurological deficit.

Spinal Dysraphism

The general group of spinal dysraphisms was classified by Lichenstein as involving the skin, underlying mesoderm, or the neural elements (9). These abnormalities are thought to result from abnormal development in the stage of caudal spinal cord formation during the periods of canalization and retrogressive differentiation.

The cutaneous lesions seen are hypertrichosis, skin nevus (hyperpigmentation), and a dermal sinus or pit. It is common for these skin changes to be associated with any of the closed neural tube defects. The presence of any one of these cutaneous manifestations should alert the physician to the presence of a closed defect. An x-ray usually shows a spina bifida and widening of the spinal canal with increased interpedicular distance.

The commonest mesodermal lesion is lumbosacral lipoma. This may be in the subcutaneous tissue alone without an intradural component; it may extend through a spina bifida, attaching to the dura, the spinal cord; or it may be continuous with an intradural lipoma. The latter condition is referred to as lipomeningocele. Depending on the intradural component, associated neurological loss can vary from none to complete paralysis. Dermoid cysts, teratomas, pilonidal cysts, and chordomas are other embryological abnormalities in this area.

When the neural tissues are involved, a meningocele or hydromyelia results. This occurs in the distal spinal cord or in the proximal filum terminale as a cystic lesion, distending the spinal cord, and is thought to be a large ventriculus terminalis. A controversial lesion that occurs during the stage of retrogressive differentiation is a tight filum terminale. This short, thick structure associated with a low-lying spinal cord is thought to be due to failure of complete retrogressive differentiation, with a tethering effect on the spinal cord, and can present with neurological deficits in the lower extremities.

VERTEBRAL ANOMALIES

During the three stages of vertebral body formation, abnormalities in the normal process result in a congenital spine defect (3,4,11,15). Congenital spinal deformities are due to one or more abnormal vertebrae with asymmetrical longitudinal growth in either the frontal or the sagittal plane. The basic underlying common denominator in all these congenital anomalies is an absence of growth potential in one or more growth plates of the vertebrae in one side of these vertebrae. Normal longitudinal growth of the vertebrae depends on enchondral bone formation at the superior and inferior end-plates anteriorly and at the articular processes posteriorly. Clinically the anomalies are categorized as those defects in which a portion of the vertebral body does not form (defects of formation) and those in which normal segmentation or resegmentation does not occur (defects of segmentation). Depending on the site of the lesion, varying types of deformities — scoliosis, kyphosis, or lordosis — are seen.

If the defect of formation is anterior, kyphosis results, if it is anterolateral, kyphoscoliosis; and if it is purely lateral, scoliosis. Failure of formation of the posterior elements is common in the spina bifidas but associated neurological problems are more important. If the defect of segmentation is anterior, kyphosis results, if it is anterolateral, kyphoscoliosis, lateral scoliosis, posterolateral lordoscoliosis, and purely posterior lordosis are seen. If there is total nonsegmentation anteriorly and posteriorly, there is no curve, but in addition, there is no growth potential with a very short torso.

The vertebral anomalies were well described by Tsou et al. (15) and divided into four groups: (a) incomplete notochordal migration, (b) nonsegmentation of the neural arch, (c) faulty hemimetameric segmental displacement, and (d) failure of formation.

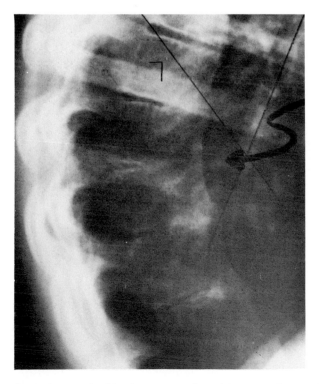

FIG. 2. Failure of anterior vertebral body segmentation with an anterior bar. Note the disc spaces posteriorly and the kyphosis due to absent anterior growth.

Incomplete Notochordal Migration

If normal notochordal migration from the centrum of the vertebral body to the intervertebral disc does not occur, with persistence of the notochord in the area of the centrum, the mucoid streak remains forming a cleft vertebra. If on the other extreme, the notochord disappears in both the area of the centrum and in the intervertebral disc, there is no segmentation anteriorly. This failure of segmentation may be partial or complete and rarely anterolateral (Fig. 2). With the absence of growth potential anteriorly and normal posterior arch growth, kyphosis results.

Nonsegmentation of Neural Arch Elements

With the migration of the mesenchyme from the sclerotome dorsally to form the neural arch, or dorsolaterally to form the transverse process and ribs, nonsegmentation at either this stage or during the stage of chondrification results in fusion of these elements. This can involve the laminae and

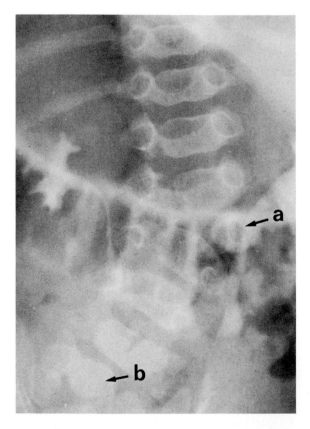

FIG. 3. Faulty heimimetameric segmental displacement. The anteroposterior x-ray shows a hemivertebra on the right in the midlumbar area L3 (a) with three normal vertebrae between it and a hemivertebra on the opposite side at the lumbosacral junction L7 (b).

pedicles, apophyseal joints, transverse processes, and ribs. When the elements of the vertebral body are involved unilaterally, the lack of growth on one side and normal growth on the other results in a unilateral unsegmented bar. This is the most malignant of all congenital vertebral anomalies. The commonest site of the nonsegmentation is in the pedicles and adjoining laminae, and the apophyseal joints (Fig. 1).

Faulty Hemimetameric Segmental Displacement

Somites form on either side of the notochord and join together across the midline, forming definitive segments which later resegment to form the vertebral bodies. If this segmentation process across the midline is abnormal —with an area where displacement of one segment occurs (i.e., the two somites join out of alignment)—half of a vertebra is left cranially and half on the opposite side caudally (Fig. 3). This hemimetameric shift results in two hemivertebrae and depending on the growth potential of these hemivertebrae, a balanced or progressive curve can result.

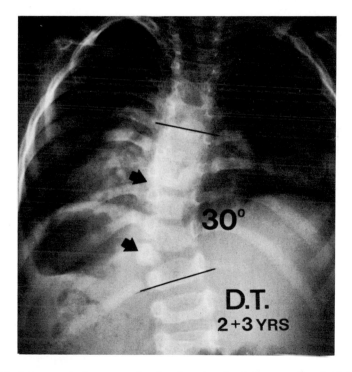

FIG. 4. D.T. Anteroposterior x-ray showing two hemivertebrae on the right. The upper hemivertebra is not separated from the vertebra above it; thus no increased growth is present on the left, and no curve progression is expected. The lower hemivertebra is separated from the vertebra above and below it and so additional growth potential exists with expected progression.

Failure of Vertebral Body Formation

The most common type of abnormality seen is a hemivertebra, where the contralateral centrum fails to form. This involves the centrum, neural arch, transverse process, and rib. This lesion probably occurs at the mesenchymal stage, with complete absence of development of one somite or "regression" of the somite at a later stage. This would give a normally developed somite on the opposite side with the resulting development of half a vertebra (Fig. 4). The theories proposing that this lesion occurs later, during chondrification or ossification, do not explain the absence of the vertebra and its processes on one side. The resulting hemivertebra can be very small (a "microvertebra"), or it may be much larger. The most minor degree of failure of formation is a wedge vertebra, with only a portion of the contra-

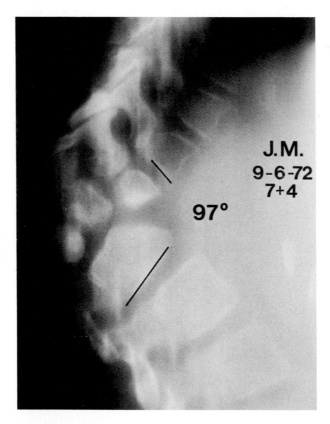

FIG. 5. J.M. Lateral laminogram at the apex of the congenital kyphus. There are three dorsal hemivertebrae which are all very small (microvertebrae). Note the bone anterior to the spinal cord, causing the cord to be sharply angulated over this knuckle of bone. In this case, the 7-year-old boy presented with early spinal cord compression and increased deep tendon reflexed and a positive Babinski sign.

lateral side not developed. Depending on the exact location of this hemi-vertebra, scoliosis or kyphoscoliosis results.

The ventral vertebral body may fail to form, resulting in a dorsal hemi-vertebra (Fig. 5). There is thus a normal dorsal centrum plus posterior elements; with this abnormal posterior growth and absent anterior growth, kyphosis results. It is thought that this anomaly either occurs during the mesenchymal stage and no mesenchyme streams ventral to the notochord, or, more likely, a normal mesenchymal body occurs with chondrification. The anterior portion of the ossification center for the vertebral centrum does not develop with a normal posterior ossification center in the centrum and thus a dorsal hemivertebra. These dorsal hemivertebrae are important as they can be multiple, lead to severe kyphosis, and cause a neurological deficit.

The prognosis for the patient with lateral hemivertebrae depends on the imbalance in the growth potential. If the hemivertebra is fused partially or completely to an adjacent vertebral body, no abnormal growth potential exists on that side and so a progressive curve does not occur. If the hemivertebra is not fused to the vertebral body and is multiple on one side, there is gross discrepancy in the growth potential with the possibility of a progressive curve (Fig. 4).

SUMMARY

These abnormalities of development are important to the neurosurgeon and orthopedic surgeon as many of them exhibit malformations of both the neural tissue and the vertebral column. They are easy to diagnose. The more important lesions are those that, with progression, can lead to neurological deficits: (a) A dorsal hemivertebra with progressive kyphosis. The spinal cord is stretched over the knuckle of the hemivertebra with cord compression and paralysis (Fig. 5). Both (b) diastematomyelia and (c) the tethered spinal cord lesions due to a tight filum terminale or lumbosacral lipoma result in failure of normal ascension of the spinal cord with a traction lesion of the spinal cord and neurological deficits in the lower extremities and bladder. Although the spinal cord has reached its "adult" position by birth or shortly thereafter, if it is under traction the normal changes in the cord during flexion and extension can aggravate this tension, with neurological changes occurring years later.

Understanding the embryology of the spinal cord and vertebrae is essential to appreciating the developmental anomalies that can occur.

REFERENCES

1. Bremer, J. L. (1952): Dorsal intestinal fistula; accessory neurenteric canal; diastemato-myelina. *Arch. Pathol.*, 54:132.
2. Cohen, J., and Sledge, C. G. (1960): Diastematomyelia. *Am. J. Dis. Child.*, 100:257–263.

3. Ehrenhaft, J. L. (1943): Development of the vertebral column as related to certain congenital and pathological changes. *Surg. Gynecol. Obstet.*, 76:282–292.
4. Epstein, B. S. (1976): Embryological considerations. In: *The Spine—A Radiological Text and Atlas*. Lea & Febiger, Philadelphia.
5. Gardner, W. J. (1960): Myelomeningocoele: The result of rupture of the embryonic neural tube. *Cleve. Clin. Q.*, 27:88–100.
6. Gardner, W. J. (1961): Rupture of neural tube, cause of myelomeningocoele. *Arch. Neurol.*, 4:1–7.
7. Gardner, W. J. (1973): *The Dysraphic States—From Syringomyelia to Anencephaly.* Excerpta Medica, Amsterdam.
8. Gardner, W. J. (1964): Diastematomyelia and Klippel—Feil syndrome. *Cleve. Clin. Q.*, 31:19–44.
9. James, C. C. M., and Lassman, L. P. (1972): *Spinal Dysraphism—Spinal Bifida Occulta.* Butterworth, London.
10. Kallen, B. (1968): Early embryogenesis of the central nervous system with special reference to closure defects. *Dev. Med. Child Neurol. (Suppl.)*, 16:44.
11. Lemire, R. J., Loeser, J. D., Leech, R. W., and Alvord, E. C. (1976): *Normal and Abnormal Development of the Human Nervous System*, Harper & Row, New York.
12. Padget, D. H. (1968): Spina bifida and embryonic neuroschisis—a causal relationship. *Johns Hopkins Med. J.*, 123:233–252.
13. Padget, D. H. (1970): Neuroschisis and human embryonic maldevelopment. *J. Neuropathol. Exp. Neurol.*, 29:192–216.
14. Patten, B. M. (1953): Embryological stages in the establishing of myeloschisis with spina bifida. *Am. J. Anat.*, 93:365–395.
15. Tsou, P. M., Yau, A.C.M.C., and Hodgson, A. R. (1974): Congenital spinal deformities: Natural history and classification. Presented to the Scoliosis Research Society Annual Meeting, San Francisco.

Spinal Deformities and Neurological
Dysfunction, edited by S. N. Chou and E. L.
Seljeskog. Raven Press, New York © 1978.

Postlaminectomy Kyphosis

John E. Lonstein

*Department of Orthopedic Surgery, University of Minnesota,
Minneapolis, Minnesota 55455*

Deformity following laminectomy for excision of ruptured intervertebral discs or for the treatment of spinal stenosis is extremely rare. The most common occurrence of deformity is in children undergoing laminectomy for the treatment of spinal cord tumors. Currently, with the aggressive care of these tumors with laminectomy, excision of the tumor, and postoperative radiotherapy and chemotherapy, a large number of these children are surviving. In the past, the child was not expected to live. The attending physicians were not aware of, or did not pay attention to the problem of postlaminectomy deformity. Now, since the survival rate has increased, the children are being referred to orthopedic surgeons years later with a severe postlaminectomy spinal deformity.

INCIDENCE

The occurrence of postlaminectomy spine deformity is rare except in children treated for spinal cord tumors (2,3,5,6). Table 1 shows the incidence in four series where these children were followed for many years after laminectomy. Of the total 251 laminectomies, deformity occurred in 124 with an incidence of 49%. The actual incidence is higher in those children who survive, as a large number of children still die from the tumor. Thirty-two patients have presented to the Twin Cities Scoliosis Center with post

TABLE 1. *Incidence of postlaminectomy spinal deformation
in four series*

	No. of children		
Study	Laminectomy	Deformity	%
Haft et al. (5)	30	10	33
Tachdjian and Matson (9)	115	46	40
Boersma (1)	51	25	49
Dubouset et al. (4)	55	43	78
Total	251	124	49

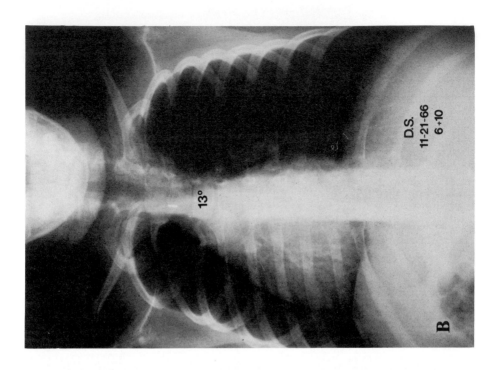

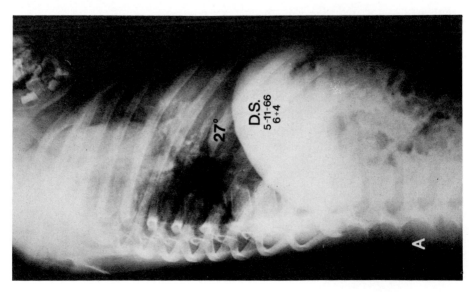

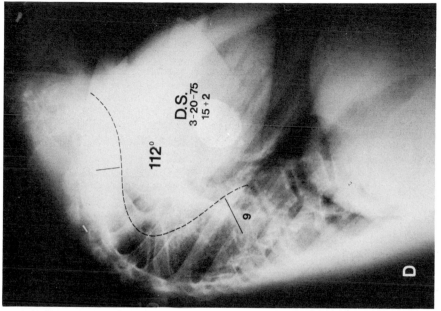

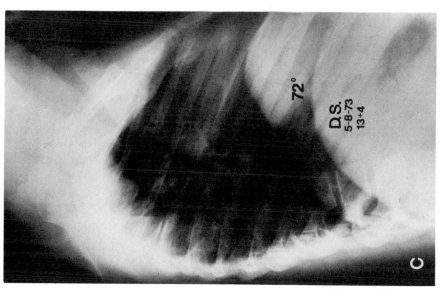

FIG. 1. D.S. This 6-year 4-month-old male underwent a laminectomy with partial excision of a spinal cord neuroblastoma and a thoracotomy 10 days later for excision of an intrathoracic extension. The area was irradiated. **A:** This preoperative lateral x-ray shows a 27° thoracic kyphosis. **B:** Anteroposterior x-ray 6 months postlaminectomy showing complete facet excision between T4 and T5 bilaterally and a 13° left thoracic scoliosis. **C:** Lateral x-ray at age 13 years 4 months, at 7 years postlaminectomy showing a 72° kyphosis—an increase of 10° per year. **D:** Two years later, at age 15 years 2 months, during rapid growth spurt, the kyphosis had increased to 112°. This 40° increase occurred in just less than 2 years.

laminectomy spine deformity, and an evaluation of these patients forms the basis of this review (7,8). All laminectomies were performed during childhood (from 6 months to 19 years) for either benign or malignant spinal cord tumors, the commonest being astrocytomas, neuroblastomas, and neurofibromas.

TYPES OF DEFORMITY

Of the three types of spine deformity — kyphosis, scoliosis, lordosis — kyphosis is the one most commonly seen following laminectomy. The deformities following laminectomy occur in the area of the laminectomy, the most common sites being the cervicothoracic and thoracic spine. Kyphosis is of one of two types: (a) short and angular; or (b) gradual and rounding. As discussed below, the extent of the laminectomy determines the type of the deformity. The kyphosis is slowly progressive during growth or it may rapidly increase during the adolescent growth spurt (Fig. 1). The kyphosis may be so severe as to cause spinal cord compression. In this case, it is usually sharp and angular. With this increasing angulation, the spinal cord is tented over the posterior edge of the vertebral body, with compression of the spinal cord and resultant partial or complete paralysis.

Scoliosis occurs much less commonly than kyphosis. It is usually in the area of the laminectomy and is associated with kyphosis. Occasionally scoliosis occurs below the area of the laminectomy, being related to the paralysis that results from the cord tumor or its treatment. In rare cases, scoliosis is the first sign of a cord tumor, progression occurring after the laminectomy (Fig. 4A).

PATHOGENESIS

On reviewing the possible causes of the deformity — including mechanical or surgical trauma, irradiation, destruction of the tissue, and neurological deficit secondary to the tumor — the mechanical cause is the most important. The posterior ligament complex, consisting of the supraspinous ligaments, interspinous ligaments, ligamentum flavum, and facet joint capsules, is the most important stabilizer of the spine. Normal muscle tone in the paraspinal muscles complement the posterior ligament complex. Gravity normally exerts a flexion of the spine in the upright position, the effects being maximal in the cervicothoracic and upper thoracic areas. The posterior ligament complex and spine extensor muscles normally counteract this flexion. With a laminectomy there is removal of the spinous processes, the inter- and supraspinous ligaments, laminae, and ligamentum flavum, and partial or complete removal of the facet joints. With removal of the posterior supporting structures, the posterior stability is lost and the normal flexion force produces kyphosis.

The facet joints are very important in determining the development of kyphosis. If the laminectomy is diagrammatically represented using the technique of Dubousset et al. (4), a correlation between the facet integrity and deformity is found. A normal spine is represented in Fig. 2A. Vertebral bodies with intact spinous processes and pedicles are seen. The facet joints are represented by two parallel lines connecting the vertebral bodies on each side. In Fig. 2B a laminectomy is shown with the spinous processes removed. When the facet joints are completely removed, no line is drawn; and when there is partial removal, a single line is drawn. By using these diagrams, a correlation between the laminectomy and the deformity is found when the initial x-rays at the time of laminectomy are evaluated. (An anteroposterior x-ray was used to draw this diagram.) When the facet joint is completely removed at one level, gross instability results, with maximum angulation at that level. A sharply angular kyphus results, with the intervertebral foramen enlarged and the disc space open posteriorly. If this complete removal is on one side only, the angular kyphus is accompanied by a sharp scoliosis with the apex at the same level (Fig. 3). If all the facets are preserved, a gradual rounding kyphus results in the area of laminectomy (Fig. 4). Thus with careful evaluation of the postlaminectomy x-rays coupled with the above knowledge, the potential deformity can be accurately predicted.

Other factors play a role in the development of the spine deformity. Radiotherapy, used for treatment of malignant spinal cord tumors, damages the vertebral growth plates, with abnormal growth resulting, adding to the deformity. Previously with asymmetrical irradiation to the spine, scoliosis resulted; but with symmetrical irradiation to the spinal cord and spine, kyphosis results. The tumor can also destroy tissue with a resulting deformity; an obvious example is eosinophilic granuloma with collapse of the vertebral body. There is also destruction of the neural tissue with slight or marked paralysis. When the paraspinal muscles are involved, this adds to the deformity. It is well known that 100% of the children with high paralysis occurring under the age of 10 develop a paralytic collapsing scoliosis (2).

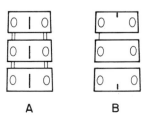

A   B

FIG. 2. A: Normal spine: vertebral bodies with intact spinous processes and pedicles. The facet joints are represented by two parallel lines joining the vertebral bodies on each side. **B:** Laminectomy. The spinous processes are removed. On the left, the facet is partially removed and a single line is drawn; on the right, the facet removal is complete and no line is drawn.

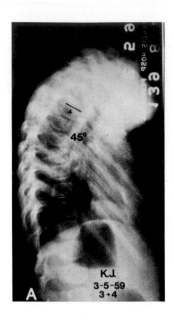

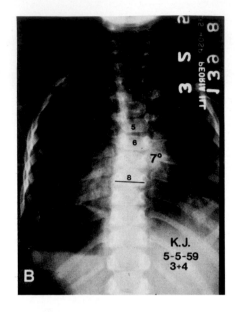

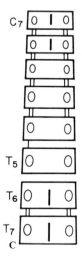

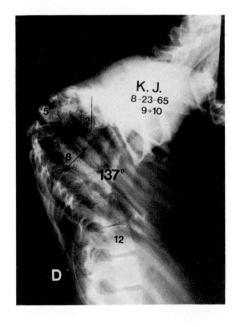

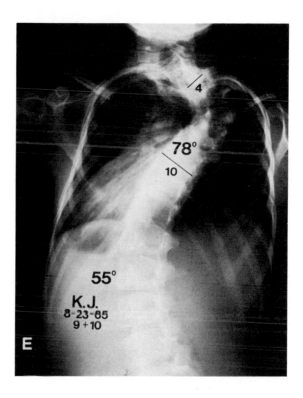

FIG. 3. K.J. This female had a laminectomy from T3 to T6 at age 20 months for excision of a neuroblastoma of the spinal cord with postoperative irradiation. **A:** A lateral x-ray at age 3 years 4 months showed a 45° kyphosis. **B:** Anteroposterior x-ray at age 3 years 4 months showed a minimal 7° right thoracic kyphosis. The absent facet joints bilaterally at the T5–T6 junction are well seen. In addition, there is no facet on the right at T4–T5. This x-ray was used for the diagram in **C. C:** Laminectomy. There is a T2–T6 laminectomy with no facets between T4 and T5 on the right and bilaterally between T5 and T6. In addition, partial facet removal occurred between T4 and T5 on the left. **D:** Standing lateral x-ray at age 9 years 10 months shows a sharp angular kyphosis measuring 137°. Note that the maximal deformity is between T5 and T6, the site of complete facet removal. The disc space is open posteriorly with an enlarged foramen at this level. **E:** Standing anteroposterior x-ray at age 9 years 10 months shows a 78° right thoracic scoliosis. Note in **C** that less stability exists on the right side as the facets are removed at two levels on this side.

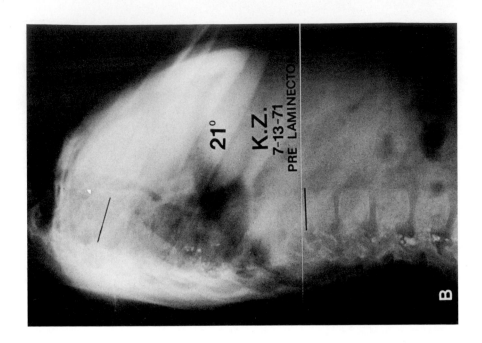

B

21°

K.Z.
7-13-71
PRE LAMINECTO...

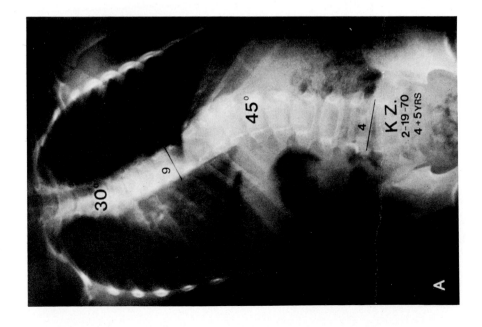

A

30°

45°

9

4

K.Z.
2-19-70
4+5YRS

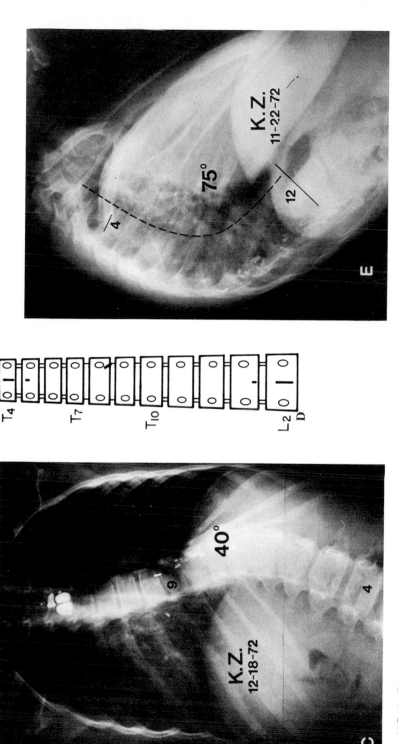

FIG. 4. K.Z. **A:** This female presented at the age of 4 years 5 months with a 49° right thoracolumbar scoliosis. This was diagnosed as infantile idiopathic scoliosis, and a Milwaukee brace was fitted. **B:** Lateral x-ray at age 5 years 10 months shows a 21° thoracic kyphosis. The child had a complaint of back pain on initial presentation as well as itching around the chest cage. A spinal cord tumor was diagnosed and laminectomy performed. A spinal cord astrocytoma was found and postoperative irradiation given. **C:** Anteroposterior x-ray at 17 months postoperation shows a 40° right thoracolumbar scoliosis. Partial facet removal bilaterally is seen between T7 and T10. **D:** Laminectomy from T6 to T12. Partial facet removal bilaterally is shown from T7 to T10. **E:** Lateral x-ray at 14 months postlaminectomy shows a gradual, rounding kyphosis of 75°.

TREATMENT

The essence of treatment of these severe deformities is early recognition and prevention. The ideal situation is for the neurosurgeon and orthopedic surgeon to confer and review the case prior to laminectomy, with the orthopedic surgeon assisting at the operation. Except for the excision of dumbell tumors (e.g., neurofibromas) the facet joints do *not* have to be removed for adequate treatment of the cord tumor. The facet joints are preserved whenever possible owing to their important role in providing spine stability. Postoperatively the child is carefully followed by the orthopedic surgeon. The immediate postoperative anteroposterior spine x-ray is examined, and the diagrams (as described above) are drawn with a potential prognosis of the deformity being made. With careful follow-up, the first sign of the deformity is found and a Milwaukee brace fitted at this time. With a long or very wide laminectomy, the onset of the deformity may occur early after surgery, and a brace should be promptly fitted to control the deformity. *This fitting should not be delayed.* If bracing is begun when the kyphosis is severe or very sharp, it fails and the kyphosis progresses inside the brace.

Since the institution of aggressive treatment of spinal cord tumors, the pessimistic outlook of the past has changed. The attitude whereby no spine treatment is rendered because the child has a malignant tumor and thus is going to die from the sequelae of the tumor must be discarded. Early referral for evaluation of the spine deformity is essential, as at this stage nonoperative treatment is still possible. With delay in referral or a late referral, bracing is impossible; the deformity at this point is more severe, and possible complications are common.

When the deformity progresses within the brace, a spine fusion should be performed. The only exception to this today is in cases where the prognosis for life is extremely poor owing to a very active or malignant spinal cord tumor.

The fusion may be performed posteriorly or anteriorly. There is only a small amount of bone surface available posteriorly after a wide laminectomy on which to attach a fusion; a posterior fusion is thus difficult. In an area of kyphosis, the fusion mass is under distractive forces, with a resultant high likelihood of pseudarthrosis. The surgical approach should thus be anterior. With a transthoracic exposure of the spine, all the discs are removed (the correction being obtained at each disc space) and the spine is fused. For a gradual, rounding kyphus an inlay strut graft is used, combined with packing disc spaces with rib or iliac cancellous bone. With a severe angular kyphosis, the rib or fibula is placed in the weight-bearing line of the spine with anterior strut grafting; in addition the disc spaces are packed with bone. In addition, posterior fusion is performed when possible to supplement the anterior fusion. With late presentation, preoperative correction with halofemoral traction is necessary before fusion is performed. With the complication of spinal cord compression, anterior transthoracic spinal cord decompression is necessary in addition to an anterior spine fusion.

SUMMARY

Postlaminectomy deformity occurs in 50% of children undergoing laminectomy for spinal cord tumors; the commonest deformity is kyphosis. Mechanical factors are the most important in the development of kyphosis, with the integrity of the facet joints being of paramount importance. With the aggressive treatment of spinal tumors, more children are surviving with these tumors and a pessimistic outlook is not warranted. Observing the deformity progressing does not constitute treatment, and early referral to an orthopedic surgeon is necessary for early bracing to control the deformity. These means of preventing deformity — early referral plus preservation of facet joints wherever possible — are essential. If surgery is necessary for progressive or severe kyphosis, the anterior approach is mandatory, with thorough excision of disc spaces and anterior spine fusion.

REFERENCES

1. Boersma, G. (1969): *Curvatures of the Spine Following Laminectomies in Children.* Born, Amsterdam.
2. Brown, H. P. (1972): Spine deformity subsequent to spinal cord injury. *Orthop. Semin. Ranco Los Amigos Hosp.,* 5:41.
3. Cattell, H. E., and Lee, C. G. (1967): Cervical kyphosis and instability following multiple laminectomies in children. *J. Bone Joint Surg.,* 49A:713.
4. Dubousset, J., Guillamaut, J., and Mechin, J. F. (1973): In: *Leo Compressions Medullaires non Traumatiques de l'Infant,* edited by J. Rougerie. Massen, Paris.
5. Haft, H., Ransohoff, J., and Carter, S. (1959): Spinal cord tumors in children. *Pediatrics,* 23:1152.
6. Haritonova, K. I., Tziuian, J. L., and Ekshtadt, N. K. (1974): Orthopaedic sequelae of laminectomy. *Ortop. Travmatol. Protez.,* 11:32.
7. Lonstein, J. E., Winter, R. B., Bradford, D. B., Moe, J. H., and Bianco, A. J. (1976): Post laminectomy spine deformity. *J. Bone Joint Surg.,* 58A:727.
8. Lonstein, J. E., Winter, R. B., Bradford, D. S., Moe, J. H., and Bianco, A. J. (1977): Post laminectomy spine deformity. In preparation.
9. Tachdjian, M. O., and Matson, D. D. (1965): Orthopaedic aspects of intraspinal tumor in infants and children. *J. Bone Joint Surg.,* 47A:223.

Spinal Deformities and Neurological Dysfunction, edited by S. N. Chou and E. L. Seljeskog. Raven Press, New York © 1978.

Mechanism of Injuries to the Spine

E. Shannon Stauffer

Division of Orthopaedic Surgery and Rehabilitation, Southern Illinois University School of Medicine, Springfield, Illinois

The spinal column functions as a flexible, mobile support of the trunk and head. It consists of an articulated series of bones of specific design connected by discs, ligaments, and joint capsules. There are specific anatomic variations and range of motion functions peculiar to the 7 cervical vertebrae, 12 thoracic vertebrae, and 5 lumbar vertebrae.

In the coronal plane the overall alignment of the spine is straight, with the center of the first cervical vertebra directly over the center of the first sacral vertebra (Fig. 1). In the sagittal plane the spine has three normal curvatures: an anterior or lordotic curvature of the cervical and lumbar spines, and a compensatory posterior or kyphotic curvature of the thoracic spine. The configuration of the posterior articulations of the three anatomic regions allow specific types of motion to occur at the various areas of the spine.

In the cervical spine approximately 50% of the flexion and extension motion occurs between the occiput and the first cervical vertebra. Fifty percent of the lateral rotation occurs between the first and second cervical vertebra. The remainder of the flexion-extension, rotation, and almost all of the lateral tilt occurs between cervical three and cervical seven.

The coronal plane configuration of the facet joint of the cervical spine with slight anterior angulation produces some obliquitory rotation with any lateral tilt and vice versa; rotation of the cervical spine also, by necessity, has some lateral tilt associated with it.

In the thoracic region the vertebrae also have facet joints in the coronal plane to allow rotation and tilt. Very little flexion or extension occurs in the thoracic spine, however, owing to the length of the vertical overlap of the facet joints as well as the resistance caused by the rib cage and sternum.

At the thoracolumbar junction the facet configuration abruptly changes from the coronal configuration of the thoracic vertebrae to the sagittal position of the lumbar vertebrae. This sagittal position of the articular facets blocks rotation of the lumbar spine and allows only flexion and extension and lateral tilt motion to occur in the lumbar spine.

The areas of the spine which allow the most motion to occur normally are at maximum risk when excessive forces are applied to the spine and thus are

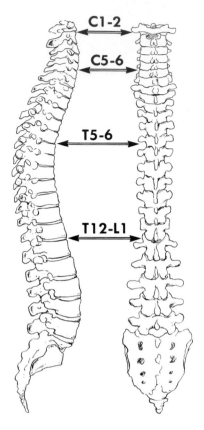

FIG. 1. Lateral and posterior views of the spinal column demonstrating the normal curvatures of the spine and the four levels that most frequently suffer fractures and dislocations.

the areas most likely to fracture. These areas specifically are: the occipito-cervical junction at C-1/C-2; the midcervical spine at C-5/C-6; and the thoracolumbar junction at T-11, T-12, and L-1 (Fig. 1).

ETIOLOGY OF SPINAL INJURIES

The etiology of 1,905 patients with spinal injuries admitted to Rancho Los Amigos Hospital for treatment over a 10-year period consisted of automobile accidents (43%), gunshot wounds (20%), falls (12%), diving and surfing (8%), motorcycle accidents (6%), and miscellaneous (11%). Automobile accidents and gunshot wounds accounted for approximately two-thirds of all injuries (Fig. 2).

MECHANISM OF INJURY OF CERVICAL FRACTURES AND DISLOCATIONS

Flexion-Rotation

The most common injury causing fractures and dislocations of the cervical spine is a flexion-rotation force, which may produce pure subluxation, dis-

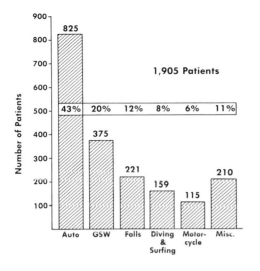

FIG. 2. Etiology of spinal fractures and dislocations causing significant neurologic injury.

location or fracture of one or both facet joints, and a dislocation of the vertebral body through the disc or a fracture through the vertebral body. With a rotational force added to the flexion force sufficient to dislocate one facet and leave the contralateral facet in the located position, the vertebral body sublexes 20–30% anterior on the vertebral body beneath it. If the flexion force is sufficient to dislocate both facets so that both inferior facets are locked anteriorly to the superior facet of the lower vertebra, the body is displaced at least 50% forward on the inferior vertebra. Oblique films are often necessary to diagnosis accurately the unilateral facet dislocation (9). With facet dislocations the spinal cord may escape injury or suffer permanent neurologic damage. The nerve roots tranversing the neural foramina at the level of injury are frequently injured with a temporary radiculopathy, and demonstrate slow, progressive recovery following reduction.

Axial Load

Axial load, or compression forces, caused by diving head-first into a shallow pool frequently produces a burst fracture of the midcervical region involving the C-5 vertebral body. This axial load may produce fractures of the posterior elements. With the axial load burst fracture the spinal cord usually sustains severe damage, and a high percentage of these patients have complete quadriplegia due to the impact of the comminuted vertebral body fragments into the neural canal causing damage to the spinal cord (Fig. 3).

Extension

Because of the strength of the anterior longitudinal ligament of the configuration of the dorsal elements, extension forces usually cause only minor

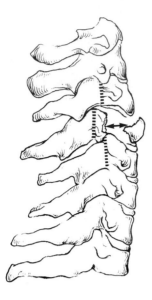

FIG. 3. Axial load burst fracture of C-4 vertebral body with protrusion of posterior portion of vertebral body into the neural canal.

fractures of the laminae and occasionally produce an avulsion of the anterior superior or inferior margin of the vertebral body. Rarely do these patients suffer injury to the spinal cord during the first four decades of life.

As one reaches the seventh decade of life, the cervical neural canal becomes progressively more narrow owing to hypertrophy of osteophytes around the narrowed intervertebral discs and thickened ligamentum flavum posteriorly. An extension force applied to the cervical spine (e.g., falling forward and landing on the forehead with the neck extended) frequently produces a momentary pincer-type injury to the spinal cord causing an incomplete quadriparesis of the central cord syndrome type, or a complete quadriplegia in the late middle-aged person without any radiological evidence of fracture or dislocation of the cervical spine (6,7).

THORACIC SPINE

The most common fractures of the thoracic spine are pathological compression fractures due to osteoporosis and are of no serious importance and rarely demonstrate neurologic deficit (Fig. 4). Severe translation forces, however, may disrupt the midthoracic spine at the T-5, T-6, and T-7 levels. The magnitude of these forces usually causes physical transection of the spinal cord in the tight neural canal resulting in permanent, complete paraplegia.

Flexion rotational forces at the thoracolumbar junction usually cause tearing of the posterior innerspinous ligaments, a fracture of one facet which carries down through the vertebral pedicle and body with a dislocation of the contralateral facet. This was described by Sir Frank Holdsworth as a "slice

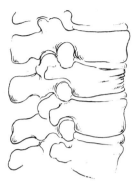

FIG. 4. Compression fracture of thoracic vertebra without dislocation or impingement on neural canal.

fracture." The superior vertebra and the superior "slice" of the fractured vertebra displace forward on the inferior portion of the fractured vertebra (Fig. 5). This is very unstable owing to disruption of both the anterior and posterior spinal column, and the patients frequently have severe neurologic damage to the spinal cord and cauda equina (3,4).

Axial load injuries to the lumbar spine cause burst fractures of the mid-lumbar vertebra, usually L-2 or L-3 (Fig. 6). If there is no disruption of the posterior interspinous ligament and the posterior longitudinal interbody ligament, these injuries are usually stable. However, if there is comminution of the posterior element or if there is disruption of both the anterior and posterior element or if there is disruption of both the anterior and posterior longitudinal ligaments and fractures of the posterior elements, these burst fractures are very unstable and usually cause severe damage to the cauda equina by retropulsion of bone fragments into the neural canal. These fractures require traction, either with internal distraction fixation or halo-femoral traction for reduction.

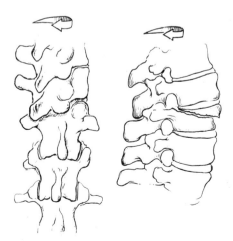

FIG. 5. Posterior and lateral views of flexion-rotation "slice" fracture at the thoracolumbar junction.

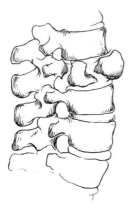

FIG. 6 Lateral view of an axial load "burst" fracture of the midlumbar spine.

SEATBELT INJURIES

If a person is subjected to severe flexion forces with the axis of rotation anterior to the vertebral column (e.g., being held stationary by a seatbelt in an automobile or plane crash), flexion-distraction forces are applied to the spine that disrupt the ligamentous bony complex either by disrupting the ligaments and allowing a dislocation of one vertebral body on the one beneath it or a pure bony fracture through the spinous process down through the pedicles and through the body (2,8) (Fig. 7). If there is minimal to moderate displacement, these fractures are stable and heal with bed rest alone. However, if there is angulation with complete disruption posteriorly, progressive angulation occurs and they require internal fixation for reduction and stability. Compression clamps posteriorly provide the most stable fixation for these injuries.

INJURY TO THE SPINAL CORD AND NERVE ROOTS

The pathophysiology of spinal cord injury is not clear. However, the damage appears to occur at the moment of impact, at which time the spinal cord ceases to function in the transmission of neural impulses. Anatomically the

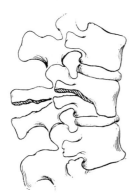

FIG. 7. Flexion-distraction fracture typical of "seatbelt" injuries.

spinal cord is rarely divided, but physiologically it ceases to function instantaneously. Persistent pressure from pieces of bone, missiles, or disc after the spine recoils back to the normal position appear to have little effect on whether spinal cord function returns. Cross-sectional studies of injured spinal cords reveal intermedullary hematoma several segments superior and inferior to the actual area of physical trauma to the spinal cord. If clinical examination reveals that the patient has an incomplete lesion, progressive recovery of varying degrees usually occurs. However, if the patient has complete anesthesia and motor paralysis distal to the level of injury and this persists for 24 hr, no functional motor recovery can be anticipated. The nerve roots which exit the neural canal at the neural foramen are frequently injured by the compression forces of the facet joints and pedicles of the injured vertebra. These injuries are more like peripheral nerve injuries, and recovery of the injured root at the site of the fracture can be anticipated in most cases.

Incomplete cord injuries may occur with partial sparring of neural function in certain areas of the spinal cord. Most incomplete injuries can be classified in one of the following categories.

In the case of *anterior spinal cord syndrome* (5), the anterior part of the cord suffers the injury, and the posterior columns are the only remaining neurologic structure intact. This patient manifests complete motor paralysis as well as paralysis of sharp, dull, and temperature discrimination, but has deep touch, proprioception, and motion sense intact.

In *central spinal cord injury syndrome* (6), only the peripheral fibers of the long tracts are spared and the patient retains perception of sensation in the sacrally innervated area. He also has intact, or can expect to recover, motor power of the sacrally innervated muscles of the toe flexors and anal and bladder sphincters.

The *Brown-Sequard syndrome* (1) describes the patient with an injury to the cord with preservation of long tracts on the opposite side of the spinal cord. This allows the patient voluntary motor control of the muscles on the contralateral side of the injury and sensory perception of the ipsilateral side.

The *posterior cord syndrome* (1), in which there is injury only to the posterior dorsal column, is rare and the patient loses only position, vibratory, and motion sense, similar to a patient with tabes dorsalis.

Nerve roots, which are present in the intraspinal canal, may be injured in addition to the spinal cord. These are lower motor neuron injuries which produce a flaccid paralysis and have a better prognosis for recovery than the injured spinal cord. In the cervical area usually only one nerve root on each side is injured at the site of the fracture, as the nerve root exits the neural foramina (Fig. 8). One nerve root level of function is very important for rehabilitation and independence training in the quadriplegic, and all efforts must be made to protect the nerve root from further injury and aid in recovery.

In the thoracic area several nerve roots transverse the injured area due to

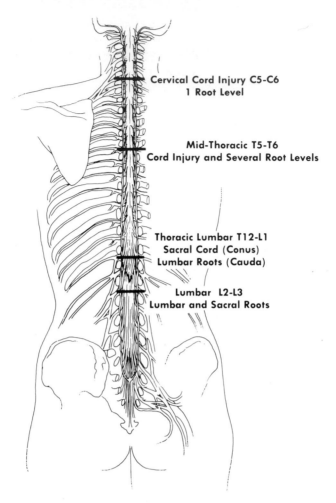

FIG. 8. Spinal cord and nerve root injuries that occur at various levels of the spinal column.

ascention of the spinal cord during development. Recovery of these nerve roots is difficult to document and is not very important since they innervate only several levels of intercostal muscles and sensation around the thorax.

At the thoracolumbar junction the spinal cord tissue consists of the sacral segments of the conus medullaris, whereas all the lumbar nerve roots (L-1 to L-5) transverse this area in the intraspinal canal. Therefore an injury to the thoracolumbar junction produces a spinal cord lesion affecting the sacral segments and a cauda equina lesion affecting the lumbar segments of motor and sensory function.

The spinal cord ends at approximately the L-1/L-2 interspace; therefore caudal to L-1, neurologic injury consists entirely of injuries to the cauda equina consisting of the lumbar and sacral nerve roots distal to the level of injury. This produces a flaccid lower motor neuron paralysis of the voluntary muscles as well as the bladder and bowel sphincter.

Knowledge of the normal anatomy and motion of the spine allows the surgeon to understand the injuries caused by forces beyond the limits of tolerance at the various anatomic levels of the spine. This understanding is necessary for a rational choice of the most appropriate therapy for the best interest of the patient.

REFERENCES

1. Bosch, A., Stauffer, E. S., and Nickel, V. L. (1971): Incomplete traumatic quadriplegia; a ten year review. *JAMA*, 216:473–478.
2. Chance, C. Q. (1948): Note on a type of flexion fracture of the spine. *Br. J. Radiol.*, 21:452–453.
3. Holdsworth, F. W. (1963): Fractures, dislocations and fracture dislocations of the spine. *J. Bone Joint Surg.*, 45B:6–20.
4. Holdsworth, F. W. (1970): Fractures, dislocations and fracture-dislocations of the spine. *J. Bone Joint Surg.*, 52A:1534–1551.
5. Schneider, R. C., Thompson, J. M., and Bebin, J. (1958): The syndrome of acute central cervical spinal cord injury. *J. Neurol., Neurosurg. Psychiatry*, 21:216–227.
6. Schneider, R. C., Cherry, G., and Pantek, H. (1954): The syndrome of acute central cervical spinal cord injury with special reference to the mechanisms involved in hyperextension injuries of the cervical spine. *J. Neurosurg.*, 11:546–577.
7. Schneider, R. C., Thompson, J. M., and Bebin, J. (1958): The syndrome of acute central cervical spinal cord injury. *J. Neurol. Neurosurg. Psychiatry*, 21:216–227.
8. Smith, W. S., and Kaufer, H. (1969): Patterns and mechanisms of lumbar injuries associated with lap seat belts. *J. Bone Joint Surg.*, 51A:239–254.
9. Stauffer, E. S., and Kaufer, H. (1900): Fractures and dislocations of the spine. In: *Fractures*, edited by Rockwood and Green, pp. 817–860. Lippincott, Philadelphia.

Spinal Deformities and Neurological
Dysfunction, edited by S. N. Chou and
E. L. Seljeskog. Raven Press, New York
© 1978.

Achondroplasia: Clinical Manifestations and Neurological Significance

Lowell Lutter

*Department of Orthopedic Surgery, University of Minnesota Medical School,
Minneapolis, Minnesota 55455*

In order to understand the clinical and radiographic manifestations of achondroplasia, a review of the developmental and radiographic anatomy of the normal spine is necessary. The normal spine evolves from one primary ossification center for the vertebral body and two centers for the arches. Overall, development is similar to that of a long bone in that longitudinal growth occurs through epiphyseal centers and transverse growth through the periosteum. One then can logically conclude that a problem in limb length is paralleled by problems in spine size. In the achondroplastic individual, longitudinal bone growth is affected but transverse growth through the periosteal contribution remains normal. Long bones are therefore short but of near-normal width. Similarly the pedicles of the vertebral column are shortened but of normal thickness. It is therefore easy to differentiate a short-trunked individual, as seen in Morquio's disease, from the short-limbed achondroplastic.

Approximately 65% of all growth-restricted individuals have achondroplasia. This is the standard of comparison and the entity about which one should be most familiar. A classic achondroplastic dwarf is short-limbed, with a slightly enlarged head and a depressed nasion. Recognition is fairly easy, but there are a number of conditions that may appear similar to achondroplasia. Radiographs can be of help in confirming the diagnosis since spine and pelvis x-rays are diagnostic in the achondroplast. In this condition the lumbar interpedicular distance in the newborn narrows or is unchanged throughout the lumbar area. This is in contradistinction to the gradual increase in interpedicular distance in a normal infant. As the achondroplastic child develops the interpedicular distance becomes narrower, and during adulthood there is a marked constriction of the lumbar spinal canal, particularly in the more caudal areas. Therefore the essential feature of the achondroplastic lumbar spine is a progressive narrowing of the intraspinal canal as one proceeds toward the sacrum. If this finding is not present, the diagnosis must be questioned. Other characteristic radiographic findings include a concave posterior border of the lumbar vertebral bodies with

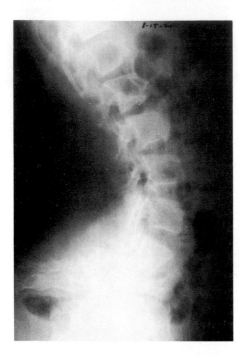

FIG. 1. Typical achondroplastic spine. Note the concave posterior lumbar bodies and the nearly equal vertebral body/disc ratio in the low lumbar area.

slightly concave dorsal edges (Fig. 1). In addition, in many areas in the achondroplast there is a relative increase in the proportion of cartilage compared to bone. This gives the disc space an increasingly widened appearance. In the normal nonachondroplastic spine the ratio of vertebral body to disc is approximately 3:1. In the achondroplast the ratio is almost 1:1. Finally, regional undergrowth may give rise to "pointed" vertebral bodies. This is especially prominent in the thoracolumbar area and may be confused with Morquio's disease. Other specific radiographic findings of achondroplasia include square-shaped ilia and a distinctive pelvis; the absence of coxa vara and epiphyseal change are of further help in confirming the diagnosis (Fig. 2).

Specific anatomic changes within the achondroplastic spine are the basis of many of the problems seen with these individuals. The first group of variations are intrinsic since they are present in all achondroplasts. These include interpedicular distance, pedicle thickness, size of the inferior facets, diameter of nerve root foramina, and intraspinal cross-sectional area. In an autopsy specimen the measured interpedicular distance of an achondroplast was noted to be approximately 40% smaller than an age-matched nonachondroplastic control (Table 1). A review of the literature, in which there are comparisons of indirect radiographic measurements, leads to a similar conclusion. It appears that pedicle thickness is the culprit (Table 1). This is further demonstrated in Fig. 3, where much of the decreased inter-

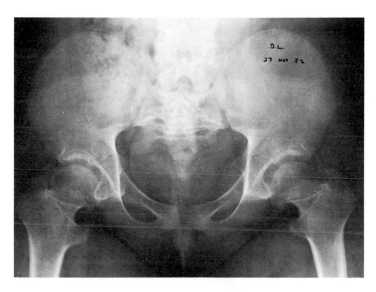

FIG. 2. Achondroplastic pelvis. Note the square-shaped ilia and the absence of coxa vara with normal epiphyses.

pedicular distance is related to thick pedicles encroaching on the intraspinal canal.

Inferior facet hypertrophy may also narrow the spinal canal, further decreasing the available space. In addition, measurement of nerve root foramina in the achondroplast reveals a decrease in size of approximately 0.2 mm at all levels when compared to similar normal spines, supporting the concept of foraminal stenosis as well as canal stenosis (Table 2). In subjecting the cross-sectional area of the spinal canal to geometric analysis, we found that the area available was approximately 40% smaller in the achondroplast (Table 3). These measurements demonstrate what has been implied radiographically, i.e., that there is decreased space available in the entire lumbar canal in the achondroplast.

In the average-sized nonachondroplastic normal spine, there is space available for the spinal cord, cauda equina, and conus medullaris, although there is a certain safety factor before encroachment on the spinal canal produces symptoms (Fig. 4). In the achondroplastic spine the contents nearly fill the canal, with only a minimal margin of safety available before further loss of this space results in neurologic symptoms (Fig. 3).

There are other anatomic factors which may develop in the achondroplastic that can be considered extrinsic. Often these result in a further loss of space, not infrequently nudging a compromised neurologic system past the recoverable stage. The extrinsic factors include disc protrusion, degenerative arthrosis, and kyphosis. In the literature, multiple disc protrusions

TABLE 1. *Transverse distances of the lumbar spine in achondroplastic and age-comparable normal spine*

| | Transverse distance (cm) | | | | | |
| | Outside (A–A¹) | | Inside (B–B¹) | | Pedicle thickness $\left(\dfrac{(A\!-\!A^1) - (B\!-\!B^1)}{2}\right)$ | |
Site	Achon.	Control	Achon.	Control	Achon.	Control
L1	4.2	3.6	1.9	2.8	2.3	0.8
L2	4.4	3.8	2.0	2.3	2.1	1.5
L3	4.5	3.8	1.6	2.4	2.9	1.4
L4	4.3	4.3	1.7	2.5	2.6	1.8
L5	4.2	4.6	1.6	2.6	2.6	2.0

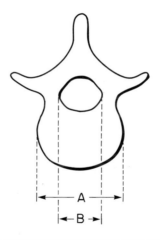

Note the absence of progressive widening in the more caudal segments in the achondroplast.

have been stated to be an important element in spinal encroachment. This factor has probably been overemphasized. In the achondroplast myelograms are usually interpreted as demonstrating multiple bulging discs. Certainly in some cases the acute onset of symptoms, especially if pointing to specific nerve roots, can be due to a disc herniation, but the idea of disc protrusion as a common cause of neurologic symptoms is uncertain. Unfortunately, a lumbar canal stenosis is often myelographically interpreted as a disc protrusion. Almost every myelographic study in an achondroplast shows

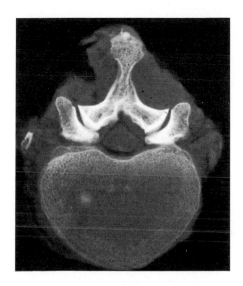

FIG. 3. Transverse section through an achondroplastic lumbar spine. Note the decreased intraspinal space when compared to Fig. 4.

evidence of scalloping on the lateral and anteroposterior views (Fig. 5). This is a manifestation of abnormal anatomy and is not necessarily a reflection of multiple disc herniations.

Degenerative arthritis in the older achondroplast, as in the nonachondroplastic patient, may produce spinal stenosis, resulting in claudication-like symptoms. Kyphosis is the third extrinsic factor. All newborn achondroplasts have a mild kyphosis of the lumbar area, producing a "bullet"-type vertebra at the thoracolumbar junction. Once the achondroplast stands and becomes ambulatory, there is a transition from a kyphotic to a lordotic configuration. In a small but important percentage of achondroplasts, the thoracolumbar kyphosis persists, and with growth there can be gradual progression (Fig. 6). These patients must be followed closely, and if the kyphosis does not diminish after ambulation, treatment with a Milwaukee brace should be instituted. In the case of progression, fusion anteriorly and

TABLE 2. *Neural foramina size in an achondroplastic and an age-comparable normal lumbar spine*

	Neural foramen size (cm)	
Site	Achondroplast	Control
L1	0.35	0.6
L2	0.22	0.5
L3	0.3	0.55
L4	0.3	0.4
L5	0.2	0.4

Note the generally smaller foramina at all levels in the achondroplast.

TABLE 3. *Spinal cross-sectional area in the achondro-plastic and age-comparable lumbar spine*

| Site | Spinal cross-sectional area (cm²) | |
	Achondroplast	Control
L1	1.29	3.35
L2	1.23	2.45
L3	1.1	2.26
L4	0.84	1.94
L5	0.77	2.84

Note the decreased available space at all levels in the achondroplast.

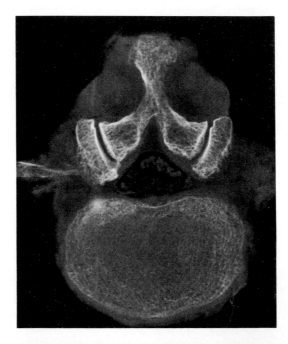

FIG. 4. Transverse section through nonachondroplastic lumbar spine; age comparable to that in Fig. 3.

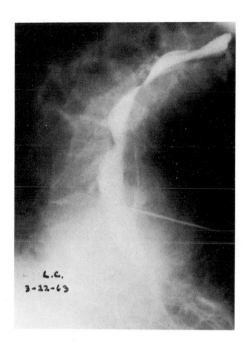

FIG. 5. Myelogram of achondroplastic dwarf. Note the false impression of multiple bulging discs, which on careful analysis is due to a constricted canal and vertebral scalloping.

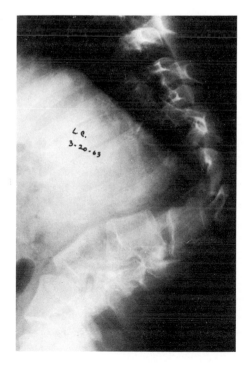

FIG. 6. Adult achondroplastic spine with severe kyphosis.

posteriorly is recommended. If neurological symptoms and signs are present, one must consider anterior decompression and fusion plus a posterior fusion. It must be emphasized that a decompressive laminectomy in a patient with such kyphosis is contraindicated. This weakens the skeletal stability posteriorly and aids progression of the kyphosis.

CLINICAL MATERIAL

We reviewed the literature and analyzed a group of 42 achondroplastic dwarfs with neurologic symptoms who had undergone spinal surgery (Table 4). In many of these patients the symptoms may have begun in childhood and usually were manifest during the teenage years or early adulthood. We classified these patients according to four modes of presentation of their neurological symptoms (Table 5).

Type I: Insidious Onset

In the type I cases symptoms of muscle weakness in the legs are insidious and intermittent. Later the paresis is coupled with paresthesias, sciatic pain, and loss of bladder control. In our study all such patients had a progressive or fixed neurologic deficit before surgery, and a large percentage of cases exhibited a kyphosis. The results of surgery in this group reveal that the vast majority remain neurologically impaired or are worsened following the surgical decompression. Significant improvement seems to be rare. The progressive neurological deterioration in this type is believed to be a consequence of mechanical compression of the cauda equina.

Type II: Intermittent Claudication

In the type II patients intermittent vague lower-extremity neurological symptoms such as pain, paresthesias, or weakness are associated with physical activity. Mechanical factors may play a role in these patients, but more likely the problem is one of transient ischemia of the cauda equina. In this group it is reasonable to assume that unless a permanent deficit occurs the surgical result will be good. All type II patients in our study underwent surgery before permanent long-tract signs occurred, even though the patients were experiencing considerable difficulty with ambulation. The surgical outcome in this group was much better than that in type I.

Type III: Disc Protrusion

Disc herniation can occur in the achondroplast. This is especially true in cases where there are symptoms and signs of radicular compression. Our series had a limited number of patients; and although the surgical results

TABLE 4. *Clinical features and operative results in 42 achondroplastic dwarfs who underwent spinal surgery*

Case	Age	Sex	Symptoms	Examination	Surgery & results
1. Vogel & Osborne: case 7	46	M	Insidious onset of loss of muscle strength. Paraplegia after 10 yr. Cramps with walking. Pt. bedridden. Urinary incontinence.	Complete paralysis of legs. Increasing sensory loss, proximal thighs to toes. Minimal kyphosis.	T10-L1 laminectomy. Improvement in bladder function to normal. Motor power increased, ambulating with crutches.
2. Vogel: case 9	21	F	Gradual progression of leg weakness	Paralysis of legs with spasticity. Ankle clonus bilateral. Decreased active motion. Poor sensation in all modalities. Kyphosis 90°.	T12-L2 laminectomy, after 3 months of traction without improvement. Flaccid paralysis developed postop. Surgery redone for hematoma. Pt. never regained preop status.
3. Handcock & Phillips: case 2	63	M	Acute onset of loss of use of legs and back. Progressive weakness until wheelchair bound. Pt. incontinent later.	Ankle and knee reflexes absent. Flaccid paralysis in both feet. No left hip or knee extensors. S1 anesthesia. Kyphosis.	L1-L5 laminectomy. Dura opened. Slight motor and sensory improvement. Pt. remained in wheelchair.
4. Handcock & Phillips: case 3	53	M	Increasing lower limb weakness. Numbness in feet and weakness made worse with ambulation. Sudden loss of sphincter control.	Bilateral positive Babinski signs. Hyperactive ankle reflexes. Decreased sensation in medial part of feet, legs, and dorsum of feet. No kyphosis.	T10-L1 laminectomy. Numbness disappeared. Leg strength returned. Two years later the weakness returned as before. L1-L4 laminectomy performed giving limited improvement.
5. Handcock & Phillips: case 4	61	M	Intermittent tingling in both legs. Two years later weakness developed after walking.	Loss of hip flexion, right. Knee extensors weak on right. Knee and ankle reflexes absent. Left positive Babinski and loss of position sense in all foot digits. Minimal kyphosis.	L2-S1 laminectomy. Left limb worse. Spasm made worse.

TABLE 4 (Continued)

Case	Age	Sex	Symptoms	Examination	Surgery & results
6. Handcock & Phillips: case 5	50	F	Slowly increasing 5-yr history of stiffness and numbness. Right leg numbness. Pt. fell down stairs and had immediate paraplegia.	Positive bilateral Babinski sign. Spastic paraparesis. Joint position sense impaired. No kyphosis.	T4-T12 laminectomy. Surgery performed because there was further deterioration of the spastic paraparesis. Had no relief from this and actually had increase in deterioration, which led to a later laminectomy of T12-T5 with no improvement.
7. Handcock & Phillips: case 7	55	F	Slow, progressive weakness and numbness. Pt. could walk only a few yards without support.	No sensory impairment. Spastic paraparesis. Increased ankle and knee reflexes bilaterally. Positive bilateral Babinski. No kyphosis.	T1-L2 laminectomy. Limb power returned to normal.
8. Handcock & Phillips: case 8	38	M	Slow progressive loss of muscle strength. Progressive paraparesis. Bowel and bladder control lost.	Flexor spasm bilateral and only voluntary motion of toes. Positive Babinski. Bilateral and analgesia below L1. Hypoalgesia T11-T12. Moderate kyphosis.	T9-L3 laminectomy. Voluntary power returned to both limbs to a slight degree. Pinprick sensation regained. Bladder control regained.
9. Epstein-Mais: case 1	15	F	Spontaneous onset of pain in legs posteriorly. Relief with bed rest. Increasing weakness. Pt. unable to walk more than one block without marked amount of pain.	No kyphosis. Ankle and knee reflexes reactive. Positive Babinski on right. Left negative. Vibratory sense decreased in toes.	T12-L5 laminectomy. Motor power returned to the point where pt. could ambulate. Babinski remained on right but not on left. Pain in back decreased.
10. Garde & Mansuy	29	F	Pain in low back with right sciatic pain.	Kyphosis. Sensory level T11. Ankle and knee	T10-L2 laminectomy and disc exploration. L1-2 laminectomy.

# / Name	Age	Sex	History	Examination	Course / Surgery
			Acute onset of paralysis after lifting heavy weight.	reflexes gone.	Sensory level was less after first surgery and there was no return. After second surgery, no voluntary foot or toe muscle. Ankle reflexes remained gone as did knee reflex and sensation unchanged.
11. DeGispert-Cruz	40	M	Progression of difficulty in walking.	Knee reflexes gone. Babinski signs normal. Sensory exam decreased from L4 and L5 level down. No kyphosis.	L1-4 laminectomy. Good result with relief of symptoms and decrease in sensory loss.
12. Weber: case 1	59	M	Slow, gradual increase of paresis in both legs. In less than 4 weeks there was a progression into true paralysis.	Analgesia from the navel down with right sacral sparing. Bilateral flaccid paralysis in legs. Right ankle reflex and knee reflex gone; left was normal. No kyphosis.	T3-8 laminectomy. Six days postop there was some decrease in paresis; 7 months postop pt. walked well with a cane. At 12 months postop bladder had fully returned. Was walking approximately 10 km.
13. Weber: case 2	23	M	At 5-6 months of slowly increasing weakness in legs, right greater than left. Progression of pain and loss of function right leg. Marked difficulty with ambulation.	No kyphosis. Spastic paresis left leg. Bilateral Babinski. Right leg totally analgesic. Bilateral ankle clonus and loss of position sense.	T2-7 laminectomy. Immediately postop the patient was worse. Slowly thereafter he improved. Pain and position sense had minimal improvement. Able to ambulate with two canes.
14. Duvosin & Yahr: case 1	33	M	Intermittent low back pain with leg radiation.	No kyphosis. Bilateral ankle reflexes decreased. S1 sensory defect. Weak toe dorsiflexors.	L3-5 laminectomy. At surgery the cauda equina was seen compressed. Two years later no pain. Ambulating well with some foot weakness.
15. Duvoisin & Yahr: case 2	29	F	Progressive paraplegia of 4 yr duration. Acute episode of severe pain	Kyphosis. Flexible and fully correctable. Increased knee reflexes	L3-5 laminectomy and later L1-2. Marked ridges noted at surgery but no herniated disc. Ambulated

TABLE 4 (Continued)

Case	Age	Sex	Symptoms	Examination	Surgery & results
			with right paraplegia and left paraparesis.	bilaterally. Ankle reflexes decreased bilaterally. Positive Babinski. Decreased position sense.	with crutches, but several years later had further progression, necessitating remaining in a wheelchair.
16. Duvoisin & Yahr: case 3	5	F	Progressive weakness and pain with walking. Paresthesia with walking, relieved with rest. Had paresthesia when rising from a chair.	Increased knee reflexes. Decreased ankle reflexes. Positive Babinski. Sensation normal. Kyphosis.	Laminectomy. Bony ridge found at T10. No change in symptoms postop.
17. Duvoisin & Yahr: case 5	13.5	M	Severe kyphosis with leg weakness. Paresthesia in right leg with urinary urgency. Progressive weakness and urinary incontinence.	Kyphosis. Ankle and knee reflexes increased. Babinski positive.	Decompression with removal of T12-L1 lamina. Neurological symptoms were unchanged.
18. Alexander: case 1	44	M	Severe groin pain. Pain in legs and weakness in left foot.	Kyphosis. Spotty sensory loss. Weakness of dorsiflexion on left. Weakness of plantar flexion.	Laminectomy, L3 disc removed. T10-L1 laminectomy. Pt. had urinary retention thereafter. Strength improved with some right plantar flexion. Weakness remained.
19. Alexander: case 2	28	F	Pain in low back area. Weakness in leg.	Kyphosis, 90° with apex at T2. Decreased sensation at S2-5.	T10 to L5 laminectomy. Pain remained the same. Weakness and decreased sensation were better.
20. Spillane: case 1	40	M	Slow onset of pain in lumbosacral region and thighs. Weak foot dorsi-	Minimal kyphosis. Paresthesia in both feet and buttocks; pain.	L2-5 laminectomy. Pt. returned to work. Regained leg function. Reflexes remained absent.

Case	Age	Sex	History	Examination	Treatment / Outcome
			flexors. Bilateral footdrop. Bilateral sensory impairment.		Sensation returned to almost normal.
21. Spillane: case 2	37	F	Left foot numbness beginning ca. 9 yr prior to later symptoms. Sciatic pain and foot weakness noted.	Bilateral footdrop. Loss of ankle reflexes bilateral. Sensation below the knees impaired. Vibration sense gone. Minimal kyphosis.	Laminectomy. Left foot no power regained. Right foot moderate improvement.
22. Bergstrom: case 2	55	F	Slowly increasing back pain with radiation into right leg. Progression with increased difficulty walking and increased pain. Difficulty in urinating.	No kyphosis. Bilateral ankle reflexes gone. Positive straight leg raising bilaterally.	Hemilaminectomy L2 and L3. Improvement postop with less pain and some symptom regression. Four years later increasing symptoms and returned to wheelchair.
23. Stroobandt: case 1	33	F	Difficulty walking. Increase in paresthesia bilaterally.	No kyphosis. Ankle reflexes increased. Bilateral positive Babinski. Bilateral straight leg-raising pain.	T12-L4 laminectomy. Marked relief of symptoms.
24. deLange	47	F	Difficulty walking. Intermittent claudication and pain.	No kyphosis. Knee reflexes absent, right.	L3-5 laminectomy. Paresthesia and pain disappeared in 3 months. Reflexes returned.
25. Schreiber & Rosenthal: case 1	33	M	Acute onset of pain in hips and feet.	No kyphosis. Bilateral radiation of pain down legs when standing. Paresthesia and weakness of legs. Left knee reflex gone. Right ankle reflex gone. Decreased sensation of right little toe. Both legs weak.	L2-5 laminectomy. Very large disc fragment at L2-3. Complete relief of pain. Pt. returned to work 6 months later. At 1 year postop had full strength in legs and was free of numbness. Deep tendon reflexes were normal.

TABLE 4 (Continued)

Case	Age	Sex	Symptoms	Examination	Surgery & results
26. Schreiber & Rosen-thal: case 2	31	F	Vague bilateral hip pain, radiation into legs. Loss of bladder control. Right leg paresis.	No kyphosis. Slight anesthesia, positive right straight leg-raising. Right lateral aspect of foot anesthetic. Knee and ankle reflexes gone on right. Left ankle reflex gone. Left knee reflex present. Weakness in lower extremities.	L2-3 laminectomy. Removal of large pieces of disc intra-durally. Bladder symptoms returned 2 months after surgery. Right foot sensation returned. Pt. able to walk slowly. Some weakness persisted.
27. McCluer	51	F	Numerous brief episodes of paralysis associated with falling. Sudden onset of complete paralysis followed by some return. Severe kyphosis.	Lower-extremity motor weakness. Inability to ambulate.	T12-L4 laminectomy. No im-provement. C6-T1 laminectomy with increased spasticity and weakness. At 1 year postop (2 yr after onset) upper arm strength better. Pt. ambulated finally in a walker and wheelchair. Became independent in ambulation.
28. Grossiord	60	M	Onset of paraplegia. Previously only fatigue with walking. Five years previously had symptoms and difficulty walking; this stabilized when he used a cane. Developed constipation and urinary problems. Then be-came paraplegic.	Positive Babinski, hyperreactive reflexes. No pain. Hypoesthesia below L2.	T11-L2. No change with sphinc-ter, slowly improved motor problems.
29. Kissel	44	F	Lower extremity weak-ness. Gradually pro-	Kyphosis. Able to walk. Fatigued easily.	T8-L2 laminectomy performed. Opened dura and dentate liga-

	Age	Sex	History	Findings	Operation and Outcome
			gressive. About 1 mo duration. Unable to walk more than 40 meters due to fatigue.	Decreased muscle strength. Positive Babinski. Decreased skin sensation.	ments cut. Immediate postop paralysis. Sphincter out. Regained muscle strength. Surgeon felt procedure not success.

PREVIOUSLY UNPUBLISHED CASES

	Age	Sex	History	Findings	Operation and Outcome
30. Case 1	46	F	Gradual onset of spastic paraplegia. Mass reflex and transverse myelopathy.	Able to walk with difficulty initially, then unable to control lower-extremity muscles.	T9-L1 laminectomy. Postop paraplegia. No recovery. Paraplegia remained.
31. Case 2	38	F	Numbness in lower extremities. Gradual progression involving first one and then the other foot. Nonradiating back pain.	Ankle reflexes absent. Sensory level at T11.	T8-L3 laminectomy. Postop hyperactive reflexes. Prepatellar clonus. Pt. returned to OR, thought a hematoma present; none found. Paraplegic. Gradually gained bladder and bowel control. Able to get out of wheelchair. Left leg voluntary muscle activity returned.
32. Case 3	27	F	Weakness in lower extremity. Weakness stable.	Some scoliosis and some kyphosis. Hyperactive reflexes both knees. Weakness right ankle.	T12-L2 laminectomy. Sensation returned. No return of motor function.
33. Case 4	35	M	Right leg stiffness and weakness. Progressive loss of muscle strength. Progressive loss of bowel and bladder control. Paraplegic.	Kyphosis. Positive bilateral Babinski's. Ankle reflexes absent. Lower extremity paraplegia.	T6-L5 laminectomy. Initially no change in paraplegia. Later some sensation returned to both lower extremities.
34. Case 5	55	F	Pain in low back. Pain became constant. Worse with motion. Weakness in right leg.	Ankle and knee reflexes hyperactive. Sensation normal. Positive straight leg-raising on right.	T10-L5 laminectomy. Initial some symptom relief and gradual progression to paraplegia over longer period of time. Postop, the paraplegia remained at L1-2 level.

TABLE 4 (Continued)

Case	Age	Sex	Symptoms	Examination	Surgery & results
35. Case 6	46	F	Increasing low back pain. Urinary incontinence.	Ankle reflexes decreased on right. Knee reflexes decrease on right.	L3-5 laminectomy. Low back and hip pain less initially. Three years later the symptoms returned.
36. Case 7	60	M	Gradually increasing parethesia noted initially in feet.	Positive Babinski bilateral. Ankle and knee reflexes normal.	T10-L5 laminectomy. Slow progress but satisfactory. Pt. used one cane to walk.
37. Case 8	38	M	Weakness in both legs. Numbness in both feet. Gradual increase in these. Pain with urinary incontinence.	Decrease in knee and ankle reflexes. Weakness in quads and foot dorsiflexors.	L1-5 laminectomy. Cardiac arrest immediately after surgery and expired.
38. Case 9	33	M	Back and leg pain intermittent. Pain gradually increased and became continuous with lifting.	S1 hypesthesia. EMG: partial denervation of peroneus longus.	T12-L5 laminectomy. Pain gone, able to ambulate long distances. Complete recovery.
39. Case 10	40	F	Bilateral weakness and giving way. Progressive disability in walking.	Left ankle reflex decreased.	T12-L3 laminectomy. Slow improvement with gradual strength regained. Maintained this for 10 yr then gradual increasing quads weakness, requiring left lower long leg brace.
40. Case 11	62	M	Low back and right leg pain. Gradual progression of right leg pain, which increased with activity.	Right ankle reflex decreased. Straight leg raising without pain.	L2 hemilaminectomy, L3 partial laminectomy. Disc fragment removed. Pt. ambulated well postop and was discharged symptom-free.

| 41. Case 12 | 25 | F | Exam at age 6 was normal. Exam at 25 yr showed gradual increase of paresthesia: first left then right Paresthesia gradually increased to the point where it was associated with activity and stopped when pt. rested. | Positive Babinski. Ankle reflex on right negative. Left 2+. | L1-5 laminectomy. Pt. ambulating when discharged approximately 10 days postop with strength approaching normal. |
| 42. Case 13 | 27 | M | Acute onset of pain in left leg. Initial treatment of traction. Pt had pain with any activity. | Absent deep tendon reflexes, left leg. | L4-5 hemilaminectomy. L3 total laminectomy. Good relief of symptoms for 4 yr. Later onset of back and groin pain; symptoms recurred on the left leg. |

TABLE 5. *Classification of the modes of presentation of neurologic symptoms in 42 achondroplastic patients who underwent spinal surgery*

Author	Age	Sex	Case reference	Kyphosis	Grade
			TYPE I: PROGRESSIVE-INSIDIOUS		
Alexander	23	F	2	+	2 Multiple laminectomies
Bergstrom et al.	55	F	2	0	3
DeGispert-Cruz	40	M	1	0	4
Duvosin and Yahr	33	M	1	0	4 Returned to work
Duvosin and Yahr	29	F	2	+	3 Multiple laminectomies
Duvosin and Yahr	5	F	3	+	2 No change
Duvosin and Yahr	13	M	5	+	2 No change
Grossiord	60	M	1	0	3
Handcock and Phillips	38	M	8	+	3
Kissel	44	F	1	+	4
Lutter and Langer	46	F	1	+	1
Lutter and Langer	38	F	2	0	1
Lutter and Langer	27	F	3	+	2
Lutter and Langer	35	M	4	+	2
Lutter and Langer	55	F	5	0	2 Multiple laminectomies
Lutter and Langer	46	F	6	0	3
Lutter and Langer	38	M	8	0	1
Lutter and Langer	40	F	10	0	4
Spillane	40	M	1	+	4 Regained most function
Spillane	37	F	2	+	3
Stroobant et al.	33	F	1	0	4
Vogel	46	M	7	+	3 Some improvement
Vogel	21	F	9	+	1 Flaccid paralysis
Weber	59	M	1	0	4
Weber	23	M	2	0	3 Cane ambulation
Average age	37.0				
			TYPE II: INTERMITTENT CLAUDICATION		
DeLange	47	F	1	0	5
Epstein	15	F	1	0	3

	Age	Sex			Result
Hancock and Phillips	53	M	3	0	4 Returned to work. Redo surgery later with grade 3 result
Hancock and Phillips	61	M	4	0	2 No improvement
Hancock and Phillips	55	F	7	0	4 Limb strength returned
Lutter and Langer	60	M	7	0	3
Lutter and Langer	33	M	9	0	5
Lutter and Langer	25	F	12	0	4
Average age	43.6				

TYPE II: NERVE COMPRESSION

	Age	Sex			Result
Alexander	44	M	1	+	4 Slight urinary retention
Lutter and Langer	62	M	11	0	4
Schreiber	33	M	1	0	5
Schreiber	31	F	2	0	3
Average age	42.5				

TYPE IV: ACUTE ONSET

	Age	Sex			Result
Garde and Mansuy	29	F	1	+	2 Sensory level slightly better
Hancock and Phillips	63	M	2	+	2 Slight improvement
Hancock and Phillips	50	F	5	0	2 No improvement
Lutter and Langer	27	M	13	0	4 (then 2 four years later)
McCluer	31	F	1	+	2
Average age	44				

Scale for results:
Grade 5: Complete recovery.
Grade 4: Very good recovery, not complete.
Grade 3: Some improvement, not complete.
Grade 2: Slight improvement or none.
Grade 1: Worse.

from this group were too small to analyze, we were left with the clinical impression that the results were good, provided the laminectomy was wide enough. In these cases, since there is such limited space in the spinal canal for accommodation of the cauda equina, a bilateral hemilaminectomy should be done to assure adequate decompression of the area.

Type IV: Acute Onset

The patients of type IV are characterized by acute, severe back and/or leg pain associated with physical activity or trauma. These patients may develop an acute paraplegia, which is one of the constant dangers in this group. In all four cases in our study, the patients had mild preexisting back pain denoting some early compression, probably placing them originally in the type I category. All of these patients then suffered acute traumatic episodes with immediate paraparesis or paraplegia. All were operated on. One expired, and three had no improvement. Certainly this suggests that the compromised neural tissue had little reserve from protection from direct injury.

CONCLUSIONS

Several statements can be made regarding surgical management in achondroplasia. Lumbar surgery must include a wide laminectomy, inferior facet excision, and nerve root foramen decompression. Surgery is tedious and time-consuming. Often it should be scheduled for two stages or performed by two surgeons. Myelography in these patients is difficult and often is of little help.

Modes of symptom onset and results are as follows. Type I: insidious onset with spotty improvement. Type II: intermittent claudication. If operated early a good result should be expected. Type III: herniated disc. Prediction of results is not possible, but these cases should be treated like any other with disc herniation. A wide laminectomy must be done. Type IV: acute onset. No relief of symptoms from surgery.

OTHER PROBLEMS

Cervical involvement of achondroplasia has received little attention. A significant percentage of older achondroplasts can develop evidence of cervical root compression. This is related to specific anatomic narrowing, similar to that in the lumbar spine. Because the cervical spinal canal narrowing is not so severe and the ambulatory stresses throughout the cervical spine less, disabling symptoms are not as frequent. Treatment should initially be conservative; but if symptoms progress and long-tract symptoms and signs appear, there is a theoretical basis for laminectomy and possible fusion. We have no cases in our series that have necessitated fusion.

The brachiocephalic shape of the achondroplastic head with increased vertical dimension gives a superficial outward appearance of hydrocephalus. Indeed, achondroplasts are in the 97th percentile for head size. During the first 12 months of life, when head growth is greatest, the head growth curve of the achondroplast parallels the normal growth curve even though actual measurements are greater. Only if the slope of the growth curve increases and ceases to parallel the normal curve is the possibility of hydrocephalus suspected. Air studies done in achondroplasts usually demonstrate a thick cortical mantel without evidence of obstruction. When obstructive hydrocephalus occurs, it is generally associated with a small posterior fossa or foramen magnum compromise, and often there are central nervous system signs related thereto. Treatment is decompression of the area of obstruction and possibly a shunting procedure.

Scoliosis is a prominent and yet not fully appreciated associated problem in achondroplasia. Basically the scoliosis is idiopathic in type. Seventy-five percent of achondroplasts evaluated by Langer had spine curvatures of mild degree. Curves tend to be short and are usually in the thoracolumbar area. The progression parallels that of the idiopathic curves. Milwaukee brace treatment or surgery should be applied with the same indications as an idiopathic scoliosis. It is important to apply the brace and perform surgery early since in the achondroplastic person the spinal cord within the narrow spinal canal does not readily tolerate additional compromise of the area.

Almost all achondroplasts have low back pain, which may begin during childhood. The back pain present in the achondroplast appears to be associated with a mechanical disadvantage placed on the lumbar facets owing to increased lumbar lordosis with a protuberant abdomen and buttocks. An additional factor may be the stenotic lumbar spine. A compensatory position for the achondroplast with spinal symptoms is that of "hunkering." The achondroplast develops pain when standing and prefers to squat on his haunches or "hunker." This is explained by studying the position of the lumbar canal and facets with standing. In this position the hips are extended and the lumbar lordosis is increased. Due to facet telescoping, the spinal canal space is decreased and the stress through the lumbar facets is thereby increased. With hip flexion, as in the "hunkering" position, the lumbosacral angle decreases and the lumbar lordosis is straightened. This creates more room intraspinally. By decreasing the lordosis some, the stenotic component of the canal is reduced and there is less sheer force on each facet, producing a position of more comfort.

SUMMARY

Achondroplasts have neurologic problems arising from: (a) intrinsic abnormal anatomy of the lumbar and cervical spine; (b) extrinsic anatomic changes at the foramen magnum; (c) hydrocephalus; (d) scoliosis; (e) lumbar lordosis; and (f) low back pain. Because of its potentially severe neurological complications, achondroplasia is not a benign dysplasia. Only by continued close observation of these individuals and early treatment of their symptoms can the disability of their problems be lessened.

BIBLIOGRAPHY

Alexander, Eben (1969): Significance of the small lumbar spinal canal; cauda equina compression syndrome to spondylosis. *J. Neurosurg.*, 31:513–519.

Bergstrom, K., Laurant, U., and Lundberg, P. O. (1971): neurological symptoms in achondroplasia, *Acta Neurol. Scand.*, 47:59–70.

Blau, J. N. and Logue, V. (1961): Intermittent claudication of the cauda equina. *Lancent*, 1:1081–1086.

DeGispert–Cruz, I. (1954): Complications neurological de la acondroplasia. *Rev. Clin. Esp.*, 53:127–131.

deLang, S. A. (1962): Eine Anomalie der Cauda Equina bei einer Achondroplastischen Frau. *Neurochirurgischen Abteilung*, 16:114–121.

Duvosin, Roger and Yahr, Melvin (1962): Compressive spinal cord and root syndromes in achondroplastic dwarfs. *Neurology*, 12:202–207.

Donath, J. and Vogel, A. (1925): Untersuchungen uber den Chondrocystrophieschen Zwergwuchs. *Wien. Arch. f. inn. Med.*, 10:1.

Elsberg, C. A. and Dyke, C. G.; *Bull Neurol. Inst.*, N.Y. 3:359 (as cited by Handcock, D. O. and Phillips, D. G.).

Epstein, J. A. and Malis, Leonard I. (1955): Compression of spinal cord and cauda equina in achondroplastic dwarfs. *Neurology*, 5:875–881.

Garde, A. and Mansuy, I. (1957): Compression de la queue cheval par hernie discale (L1-2) au cours d'une achondroplasie. Recuperation apres intervention. *Societe Francaise de Neurologie*, 371:374.

Grossiord, A., Guiot, G., Held, J. P., Tournilhac, M., and Besson, J. (1956): Lesion meduallaires dans l'achondroplasie role des anomalies vertebraie. *Rev. Neurol.*, 94: No. 4, 329–334.

Handcock, D. O. and Phillips, D. G. (1965): Spinal compression in achondroplasia. *Paraplegia*, 3:22–33.

Kissle, P., Hartemann, P., Barrucand, D., and Montaut, J. (1963): Compression medullaire et achondroplasie, *Rev. Neurol.*, 109: No. 5.

McCluer, S. and McElroy, Ann (1961): Rehabilitation of an Achondroplastic Dwarf with Paraplegia, *Physiotherapy Rev.*, 41:343.

Nelson, N. A. (1970): Orthopedic aspects of chondrodystrophies, the dwarf and his orthopedic problems. *Ann. R. Coll. Surg.*, 47:187–201.

Nelson, N. A. (1972): Spinal stenosis in achondroplasia. *Proc. R. Soc. Med.*, 65:1028–9.

Schatzer, J. and Pennel, G. F. (1968): Spinal stenosis as a cause of cauda equina compression. *J. Bone Joint Surg.*, 50B: No. 13, 606–618.

Spillane, John D. (19xx): Three cases of achondroplasia with neurological complications. *J. Neurol. Neurosurg. Psychiatr.*, 15:246–252.

Schreiber, F. and Rosenthal, H. (1952): Paraplegia from ruptured disc in achondroplastic dwarf. *J. Neurosurg.*, 6:648–651.

Stroobandt, G., Laterre, E. C., Vincent, A., and Cornelis, G. (1971): Compression radioculomedullaire d'origine and rachidienne chez une chondroplase. *Neurochirurgie*, 16:295–306.

Vogel, A. and Osborne, R. I. (1949): Lesions of the spinal cord (transverse myelopathy) in achondroplasia. *Arch. Neurol. Psychiatr.*, 61:644–662.

Weber, Von. G. (1953): Ruckenmarkskompression bei Chondrodystrophie, *Schweiz Arch. Neurol. Neurochir. Psychiatr.*, 71:291–308.

ADDITIONAL BIBLIOGRAPHY

Bailey, J. A. (1970): Orthopedic aspects of achondroplasia. *J. Bone Joint Surg.*, 52A:1285–1301.

Caffey, J. (1958): Achondroplasia of pelvis and lumbosacral spine. *Am. J. Roentgenogr.*, 8:449–457.

Cohen, M. E., Rosenthal, A. D., and Matson, D. D. (1967): Neurologic abnormalities in achondroplastic children. *J. Pediatr.,* 71:367.

Langer, L. D. (1977): Personal commentary.

Langer, L. D., Baumann, P. A., and Gorlin, R. J. (1967): Achondroplasia. *Am. J. Roentgenogr.,* 100:12–26.

Lutter, L. D. (1977): The spine deformity problem in patients with dwarfing disease. In: *Manual on Deformities of the Spine,* p. 108. Twin Cities Scoliosis Center, Minneapolis, Minnesota.

Lutter, L. D. and Langer, L. D. (1977): Neurological symptoms in achondroplastic dwarfs — surgical treatment. *J. Bone Joint Surg.,* 59A: No. 1.

Lutter, L. D., Lonstein, J. E., Winter, R. B., and Langer, L. O. (1978): Anatomy of achondroplastic spine and surgical implications. *Clin. Orthop. (in press).*

*Spinal Deformities and Neurological
Dysfunction*, edited by S. N. Chou and
E. L. Seljeskog. Raven Press, New York
© 1978.

Myelographic Evaluation of Curvatures of the Spine

Lawrence H. A. Gold

*Section of Neuroradiology, University of Minnesota Hospitals,
Minneapolis, Minnesota 55455*

Patients with presumed idiopathic or congenital kyphoscoliosis may have an intraspinal tumor or other abnormality as the etiology of their spinal curvature. In one series of 115 patients with intraspinal tumors (3), 31 patients had scoliosis and 17 kyphosis at the time of their initial examination. Since these figures represent highly significant numbers of patients, it is extremely important that, prior to surgical intervention to correct the spinal curvature, intraspinal tumors or other significant abnormalities be excluded. Myelography (1) is the best way to exclude intraspinal pathology. Obviously, those patients with a spinal curvature and evidence of neurological motor and/or sensory deficit require a myelogram. Also those scoliosis patients who complain of pain or muscular spasms should have a myelogram. Patients who present only with a spinal curvature, who are otherwise neurologically intact, and who have an apparent etiology for their scoliosis do not require a myelogram. There are some patients in whom the decision of whether to order a myelogram is unclear. In these cases the decision is a clinical one based on judgment, knowledge, and experience.

MYELOGRAPHY

Myelography in patients with spinal curvatures should be performed via a lumbar puncture with a 19-gauge short-beveled disposable needle. The puncture is usually made over the third lumbar vertebra, with the puncture being precisely in the midline. After withdrawing 5 to 10 cc cerebrospinal fluid (CSF) for laboratory examination, Pantopaque (ethyl iodophenyl-undecylate preparation) is placed in the lumbar subarachnoid space. There is considerable variability in the volume of Pantopaque utilized. As a rule, enough contrast medium is utilized to outline completely and satisfactorily the subarachnoid space and spinal cord in the areas of abnormal curvature with the patient upright at approximately a 45° angle. The volume of contrast utilized may range from 36 to 80 cc, although in a few cases as much as

120 cc contrast medium has been used. In those patients in whom more than 45 cc Pantopaque is used, approximately 25 cc CSF should be withdrawn prior to instilling the contrast material. Patients with large lumbar thecal sacs require more contrast medium than those with normal or small lumbar sacs.

Once the instillation of Pantopaque is complete, spot films are taken in the anteroposterior (AP) position and both oblique projections, covering the entire Pantopaque column. Cross-table lateral films are performed, and the patient is then placed in the head-down position. Complete cervical and upper thoracic films are done in the same manner. If the patient has such a large lumbar sac it would require an obviously excessive amount of contrast medium to fill it, then arbitrarily 60 cc contrast is used and the patient is placed in the head-down position. This way, the entire cervical and thoracic areas can still be completely filled. This alternative method is useful if the area of interest is the thoracic region; however, if the lumbar area is of interest, the lumbar sac must be completely filled.

At the end of the procedure, the Pantopaque is completely withdrawn, the needle removed, and the patient returned to his room with instructions to remain flat in bed for at least 24 hr.

Use of an inadequate amount of contrast medium and/or failure to take coned-down oblique spot films at all levels may result in intraspinal pathology being overlooked. An adequate amount of Pantopaque is that amount which completely fills the dural sac at and around the level of clinical interest.

COMPLICATIONS OF LARGE-VOLUME MYELOGRAPHY

The complications associated with utilization of large volumes of Pantopaque are similar to those of routine myelography. Headaches are the major problem. Our experience is that occasionally patients complain of severe headaches, but usually the quality and duration of the headaches are no different than for routine myelography. Patients may complain of back pain, particularly with the larger volumes of Pantopaque. The patient may actually be able to point out the level of the Pantopaque column as it rises in the lumbar and thoracic regions. This type of back pain is presumably related to pressure and "dragging" on the nerve roots by the large amounts of Pantopaque, which is heavier than CSF. This back pain is relieved by placing the patient in a flatter position, and it usually disappears when the contrast medium is withdrawn at the end of the study. There have been no deaths or neurological sequelae in our experience related to large-volume myelography.

DISCUSSION

In a previous paper (1) it was reported that 4 of 32 patients with scoliosis demonstrated unsuspected abnormalities. There were two patients with syringomyelia, one with diastematomyelia, and one with an intraspinal lipoma. In addition to detecting unsuspected abnormalities, myelography is important in evaluating the size of the subarachnoid space, severity of compression of the spinal cord, and the degree of block present. It should be noted that, in all cases reported (1), the spinal cord is displaced toward the concave side of the scoliosis with subsequent narrowing or obliteration of the subarachnoid space along the concavity of the scoliosis.

The neurological deficits associated with curvatures of the spine are probably related to traction and/or pressure on the spinal cord because of compression of the cord against the vertebral bodies. Hilal and Keim (2) demonstrated diminished intersegmental flow in the anterior spinal artery at the apex of the spinal curve, thereby proposing a possible vascular basis for neurological deficits in patients with spinal curvatures preoperatively and in those with postoperative neurological deficits.

ILLUSTRATIVE CASES

Case 1

Figure 1 shows frontal and lateral views of a patient with moderate idiopathic scoliosis in whom 56 cc Pantopaque was utilized. The entire dural sac up to the midthoracic region is well visualized with the patient in the semi-upright position. The spinal cord is beautifully demonstrated in both projections.

Case 2

Figure 2 shows severe scoliosis secondary to neurofibromatosis; 48 cc Pantopaque was used. The spinal cord is plastered tightly against the curvature of the spine, and there is obliteration of the subarachnoid space on the inner aspect of the scoliosis. The entire subarachnoid space and spinal cord are well demonstrated.

Case 3

Figure 3 shows frontal and lateral projections in a patient with severe congenital kyphosis, using 42 cc Pantopaque. Severe compression and a partial block is evident in the lower thoracic region. There is compression of the spinal cord against the posterior aspects of the vertebral bodies and obliteration of the subarachnoid space anteriorly on the lateral view.

Case 4

Moderate kyphoscoliosis secondary to neurofibromatosis is seen in Fig. 4; 86 cc Pantopaque was utilized. The plain films show marked scalloping

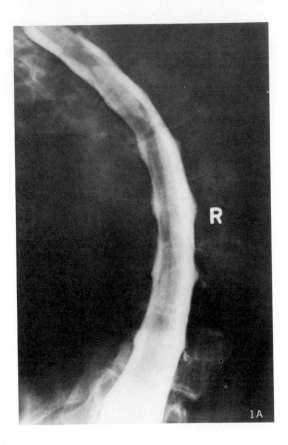

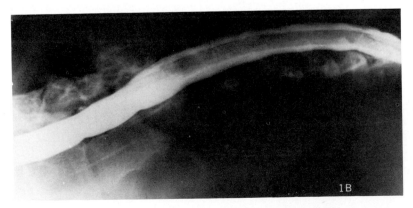

FIG. 1. Moderate idiopathic scoliosis. (From ref. 1).

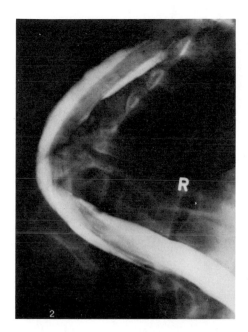

FIG. 2. Severe scoliosis secondary to neurofibromatosis.

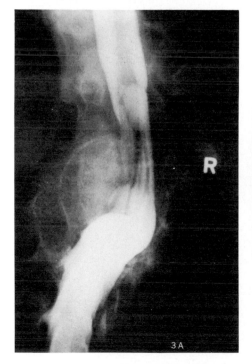

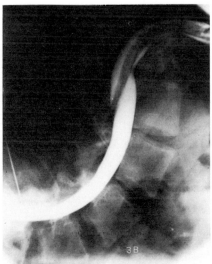

FIG. 3. Severe congenital kyphosis. (From ref. 1.)

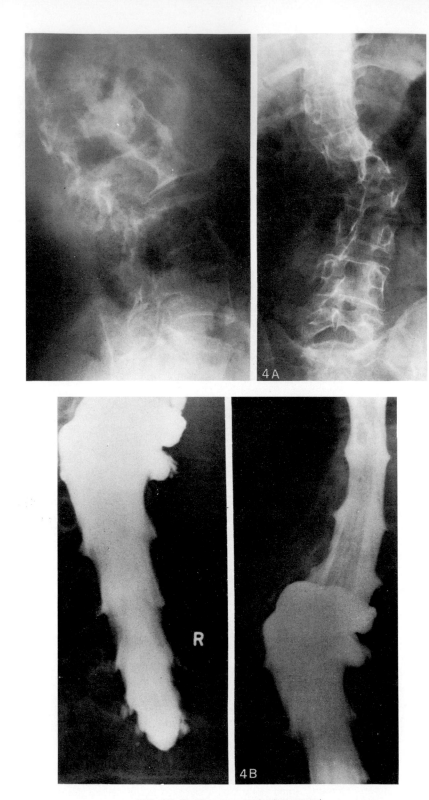

FIG. 4A–B. *(See legend facing page.)*

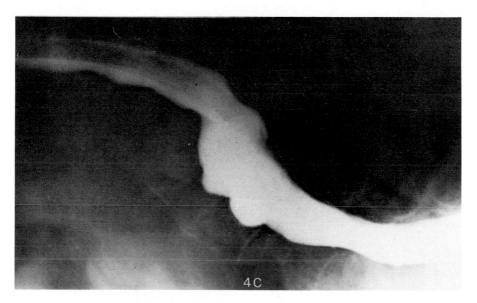

FIG. 4. Kyphoscoliosis secondary to neurofibromatosis with associated dural ectasia.

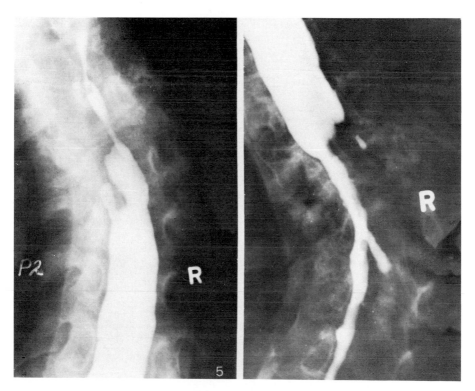

FIG. 5. Mild scoliosis in the midthoracic region. This illustrates a completely inadequate volume of contrast medium. Small tumors in the region of the curvature may be completely missed. (From ref. 1).

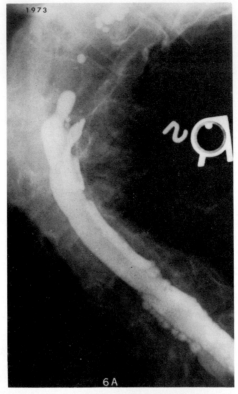

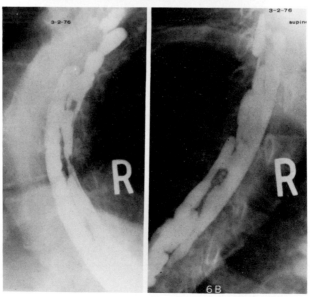

FIG. 6A–B. *(See legend facing page.)*

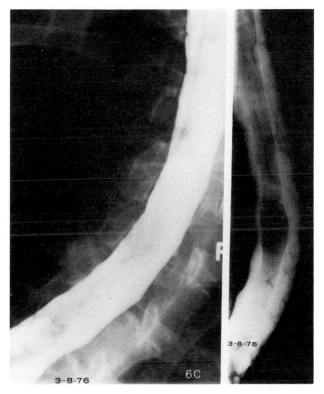

FIG. 6. Serial myelograms illustrating the necessity of a large volume of contrast medium and a tightly coned, high-kilovoltage spot film technique in order to visualize the thecal sac and spinal cord properly. The diagnosis in this case is an intramedullary arteriovenous malformation.

of the posterior aspects of L1 and L2. The myelogram demonstrates a very large lumbar sac and dural ectasia with herniation of the dura anteriorly at the first and second lumbar levels accounting for the scalloped vertebrae. The spinal cord is nicely demonstrated and is normal.

Case 5

Figure 5 demonstrates mild scoliosis in the midthoracic region. Although 36 cc contrast medium was utilized, this amount and the spot films are totally inadequate to evaluate the subarachnoid space and the spinal cord at the level of scoliosis. Small tumors or arteriovenous malformations may be easily missed with this type of inadequate study. The region of the curvature must be completely filled with Pantopaque and multiple spot films in different projections obtained. Also, spot films with very tight coning and high kilovoltage should be obtained to best visualize the spinal cord (see Case 6).

Case 6

Serial myelograms obtained from a 53-year-old female who had had scoliosis for approximately 20 years are seen in Fig. 6. Seven years prior to admission, she had an acute episode of neurological deficit with gradual improvement. She has had two previous myelograms in an attempt to visualize an intraspinal abnormality, the most recent one 6 days prior to her definitive myelogram at the University of Minnesota. She has had the recent onset of a Brown-Sequard syndrome with a sensory level at T6.

The first myelogram (Fig. 6A), performed at another hospital, is completely inadequate because an insufficient volume of Pantopague was utilized and the region of scoliosis was improperly visualized. The second myelogram (Fig. 6B) was performed 6 days prior to admission to the University of Minnesota Hospitals. Although more Pantopaque was used here than during the first examination, the amount of contrast is still insufficient. Although a supine and a prone study were performed, the diagnosis was missed and the study interpreted as normal. Besides an inadequate volume of contrast medium, tightly coned, high-kilovoltage spot films to visualize the spinal cord were not taken.

The third myelogram (Fig. 6C) was performed at the University of Minnesota Hospitals utilizing 60 cc Pantopaque. The spot film with the cones open failed to demonstrate the pathology. The subarachnoid space is well visualized, but the spinal cord is poorly seen. With a tightly coned, high-kilovoltage spot film technique, the spinal cord is beautifully demonstrated. Also well visualized is the subtle but very definite small segment of spinal cord widening at T5–T6. This indicates an intramedullary mass lesion which at surgery turned out to be an intramedullary arteriovenous malformation.

This case demonstrates that (a) sufficient Pantopaque must be utilized to fill the subarachnoid space in the region of clinical interest, and (b) that a tightly coned, high-kilovoltage spot film technique must be utilized in order to visualize the spinal cord properly.

Case 7

An 18-year-old male had a diagnosis of idiopathic scoliosis. The myelogram (Fig. 7), utilizing 60 cc Pantopaque, demonstrates an unsuspected syringomyelia involving the cervical and thoracic spinal cord. The myelogram shows diffuse and marked widening of the spinal cord shadow. Figure 7A is a lateral view in the thoracic region, and Fig. 7B is a frontal spot film in the cervical region.

Case 8

A 19-year-old female had the onset of right leg pain 3 months prior to admission. After the pain developed, she noticed progressive and severe

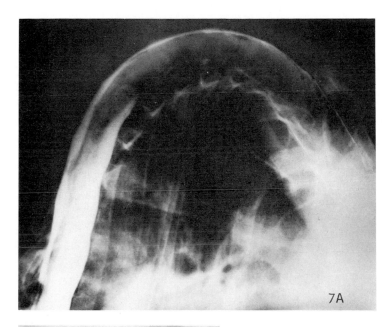

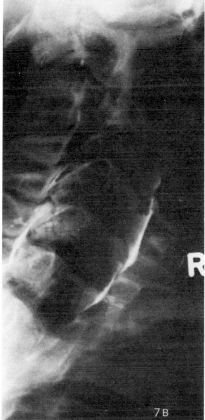

FIG. 7. The large-volume myelogram demonstrates a spectacular case of unsuspected syringomyelia in an 18-year-old male with a diagnosis of idiopathic scoliosis. (From ref. 1.)

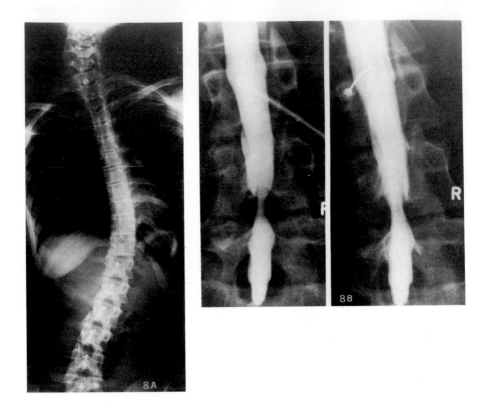

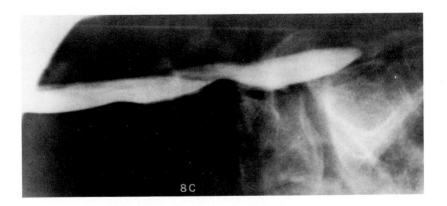

FIG. 8A–C.*(See legend facing page.)*

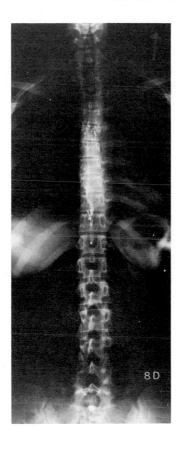

FIG. 8D. Spine films demonstrate an unusual presentation of a herniated disc with moderately severe scoliosis. The myelogram shows the herniated disc at L4–L5. After surgical removal of the disc, the scoliosis completely disappears.

scoliosis. The admission frontal spine films (Fig. 8A) show a marked lumbar scoliosis convex to the right with a compensatory thoracolumbar scoliosis convex to the left. The myelogram (Fig. 8B,C) shows a large extruded disc at the L4–L5 interspace. After surgery and removal of her herniated disc, a follow-up spine film (Fig. 8D) demonstrates a complete return to normal.

REFERENCES

1. Gold, L. H. A., Leach, C. G., Kieffer, S. A., Chou, S. N., and Peterson, H. O. (1970): Large volume myelography: An aid in the evaluation of curvatures of the spine. *Radiology,* 97:531–536.
2. Hilal, S. K., and Keim, H. A. (1972): Selective spinal angiography in adolescent scoliosis. *Radiology,* 102:349–359.
3. Tachdjian, M. O., and Matson, D. D. (1965): Orthopaedic aspects of intraspinal tumors in infants and children. *J. Bone Joint Surg.,* 47-A:223–248.

Spinal Deformities and Neurological Dysfunction, edited by S. N. Chou and E. L. Seljeskog. Raven Press, New York © 1978.

Cervical Spinal Deformity With Neurologic Dysfunction

Edward L. Seljeskog, M.D.

Department of Neurosurgery, University of Minnesota Medical School, Minneapolis, Minnesota 55455

In considering deformations of the cervical spine that may result in neurologic disability, two basic pathological processes warrant consideration. The first of these is related to intrinsic osseous pathology, with vertebral collapse and resultant spinal deformation. The second is the deformity related to ligamentous disease or injury, with related vertebral subluxation or postfracture pseudarthrosis. The former condition is basically a problem of deformity with vertebral stability, whereas the latter is a deformity related solely to spinal instability. Obviously there are cases in which there is operant a combination of these two basic factors, but an artificial classification of this sort has a practical consideration in that appropriate therapy of the two groups is quite different. In those cases that are purely related to deformity without instability, decompressive surgery is the primary mode of management. In contradistinction, for the deformities related to spinal instability and subluxation, surgical stabilization is required.

In reviewing the general etiologic factors producing spinal deformity, a number of conditions can be responsible. These are broadly categorized in Table 1. Note that within the stable spinal group are problems representing primary diseases of bone with vertebral deformation, including neoplasia, osteoporosis, sepsis, trauma, iatrogenic (postsurgical), and developmental conditions. Certainly the most commonly encountered surgical cases within this group are the problems of primary neoplasia or metastatic malignancy. Within the unstable group, trauma represents the most frequent causative factor with its ligamentous disruption and vertebral subluxation. Other unstable conditions include the loss of ligamentous support in rheumatoid disease, localized sepsis and inflammatory reaction with ligament destruction, joint instability due to sensory loss, and postsurgical instability.

UPPER CERVICAL SPINE

Stable Spine with Progressive Deformity

Among the deformities encountered in the upper cervical area, basilar invagination at the craniovertebral junction is one of the more commonly

TABLE 1. *General factors resulting in cervical spinal deformity*

Stable Spine with Progressive Deformity
   Primary diseases of bone
   Osteoporosis
   Developmental
   Neoplastic
   Posttraumatic
   Postsurgical
   Osteomyelitis
Spinal Instability with Deformity
   Posttraumatic
     Ligamentous
     Fracture with pseudarthrosis
   Postinfectious
   Rheumatoid
   Postsurgical
   Neurologic
   Developmental

encountered conditions (Table 2). Most often this deformity at the skull base is an incidental radiographic finding often found in association with other abnormalities of the area, e.g., assimilation of the atlas. In most cases there is no evident etiology, and the problem is apparently developmental in origin (8,11,14,16,20,27). In Penning's (20) classification this is referred to as basilar coarctation. In others a definite causation is documented, most often Paget's disease or rheumatoid arthritis (Fig. 1). In the former condition, bony softening around the foramen magnum allows invagination of the upper cervical spine into the occiput, referred to as basilar impression. In rheumatoid arthritis there is joint destruction, with collapse and again invagination of the upper cervical bony elements into the foramen magnum, so-called basilar erosion or pseudobasilar invagination. In both of these conditions

TABLE 2. *Upper cervical spinal deformities*

Stable Spine with Progressive Deformity
   Basilar coarctation
   Basilar impression
   Basilar erosion
   Metastatic disease
   Posttraumatic
Spinal Instability with Deformity
   Posttraumatic
     Nonunited odontoid fractures
     Atlanto-axial subluxation
     Occipito-atlantal subluxation
   Postinfectious C-1/C-2 subluxation
   Rheumatoid subluxation
   Developmental
   Posttransclival surgery

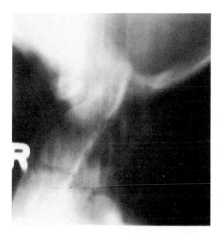

FIG. 1. Moderately severe basilar erosion (pseudobasilar invagination) due to rheumatoid arthritis. Note the significant compromise of the spinal canal and foramen magnum by the upward invagination of the odontoid process.

there exists the potential of cervicomedullary compression by the upward-projecting odontoid process. At times this deformity can be very significant, and it is surprisingly often without an associated neurologic abnormality (Fig. 2). In these cases catastrophic neurologic sequelae can acutely develop, with additional deformation of the area or following minor trauma.

When confronted with a problem of neurologic dysfunction secondary to basilar impression or basilar erosion, posterior decompression of the foramen magnum and upper cervical cord is usually the surgical procedure of choice. This allows the spinal cord and brainstem to be displaced dorsally away from the mass of the ventrally located dens. Thick arachnoidal adhesions at the level of the foramen magnum are usual, necessitating their division with microdissection, and often a generous dural graft is necessary prior

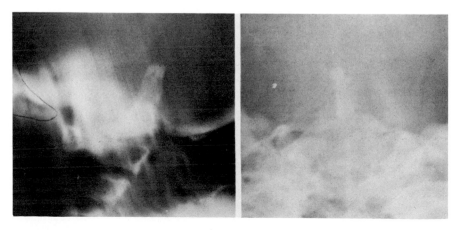

FIG. 2. Severe case of basilar erosion due to rheumatoid arthritis with its ligamentous laxity and joint destruction. Surprisingly, this patient had reasonably intact neurologic function.

to closure. In addition, there is often further compromise of the area by an associated hind brain abnormality, usually an Arnold-Chiari malformation. When there is massive upward herniation of the odontoid process, usually an anterior transoral approach for excision of the dens must be considered as a surgical alternative (22,28). Extreme care is necessary when removing this offending mass of bone since it has usually invaginated itself well into neural tissue, and injudicious maneuvers can easily result in a catastrophic surgical complication. One could also consider this type of anterior technique as a secondary procedure following posterior decompression, where there is continued neural impairment. Under most of the circumstances of an anterior or posterior decompression in this region, cervical fusion is not necessary, since in most cases the ligamentous structures of the area are intact. In the case of basilar erosion associated with rheumatoid disease, there is a combination of bony deformity and instability due to considerable ligamentous relaxation in the area. This necessitates an anterolateral or posterolateral arthrodesis of the unstable region. Usually this can be accomplished only laterally in the facet joints, since the patient has likely undergone a prior posterior decompression. A significant period of postoperative external immobilization using a halo device is commonly necessary with this lateral type of facet joint fusion.

In a similar fashion metastatic problems involving the upper cervical spine can result in progressive vertebral collapse, usually involving the second or third vertebral level (Fig. 3). Often external bracing coupled with radiation therapy is more than adequate treatment; but in those cases where there is significant and progressive angulation with neural dysfunction, anterior decompression and fusion is necessary. This is described in the discussion of the mid and lower cervical spine.

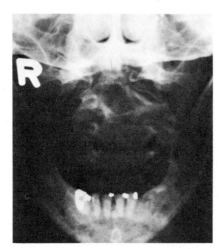

FIG. 3. Metastatic carcinoma involving the second cervical vertebra. Note the blastic character of the lesion and the collapse of the left lateral mass and its joint surfaces.

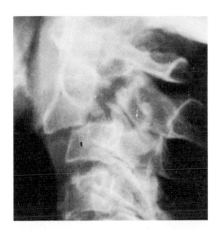

FIG. 4. "Hangman's fracture" involving a fracture dislocation through the pedicles of C-2. Despite its appearance these patients are usually intact neurologically, and the fracture usually heals well without collapse and deformity. (From ref. 25).

The final stable condition with deformity of the upper cervical spine is that of a progressive posttraumatic fracture deformity. This is an unusual condition in the upper cervical area, since most fractures are "burst" injuries and generally heal well with appropriate external support. Even the most comminuted of fractures (e.g., a severe Hangman's fracture of C-2) are not often prone to further collapse (Fig. 4). This, coupled with the larger dimensions of the upper cervical canal, often allow significant posttraumatic deformities to exist without spinal cord compression, and the need for decompressive surgery is infrequent (21,25). If so, the problem would best be managed as described for basilar invagination or metastatic C-2 deformities.

Spinal Instability with Deformity

In contradistinction to the stable deformities of the upper cervical area, problems of instability due to ligamentous disruption are much more frequently encountered. These result in deformity and neural compression due to subluxation through an intervertebral disc space or, in the case of some injuries, through a pseudarthrosis that has developed at a fracture site. The most common of these problems in the upper cervical area is that of the nonunited odontoid fracture (Fig. 5). The odontoid fracture has garnered a rather notorious reputation for developing non-union, and this is justly deserved in the minimally treated case (1,17). In our experience, however, and using more vigorous methods of closed management, the odontoid fracture can be expected to heal spontaneously in a high percentage of cases with early and adequate immobilization (23,24). In reviewing our experience for the period 1967-1976 involving 65 cases, in only two instances was there a failure of fracture healing with what was deemed to be adequate treatment. Interestingly, 12 of the 65 patients were seen late, after they had developed obvious instability and fracture non-union.

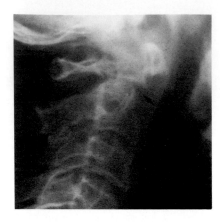

FIG. 5. Nonunited odontoid fracture with instability and anterior subluxation. (From ref. 23.)

When confronted with a nonunited odontoid fracture, with or without neurologic involvement, we advocate posterior cervical fusion using autogenous rib grafts and wiring, incorporating the laminae of C-1 through C-3 (Fig. 6). Prior to surgery the subluxation is reduced as best as possible with traction, and the operative procedure is carried out in traction in the prone position on a circle bed or other traction frame (Fig. 7). With this technique one can anticipate immediate, solid immobilization of the upper cervical area and frequently prompt resolution of the chronic neck discomfort so often afflicting these patients (Fig. 8). With this technique we have had no case of postoperative pseudarthrosis or continued instability among the post-traumatic instability problems. As an alternative, one could consider using wiring, iliac crest grafts, or possibly acrylic struts for stabilization of the area (10,15). However, our experience with the acrylic technique has been limited to cases of instability in metastatic or rheumatoid disease. Additionally, some surgeons advocate an anterior, transoral, or transcervical-retropharyngeal approach to the unstable odontoid fracture (3,6,26). This involves excision of the dens and obviously a concomitant anterior fusion of the C-1/C-2 joints. This method does not seem to offer any significant advantage over the posterior approach, and postoperative external immo-

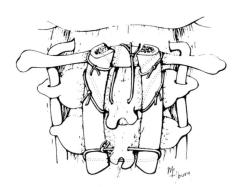

FIG. 6. C-1,2,3 posterior fusion for non-united odontoid fracture instability using rib graft struts.

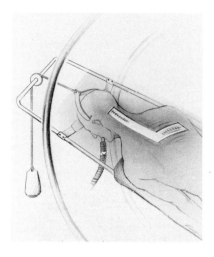

FIG. 7. Operative positioning in the circle bed for unstable upper cervical fractures using the rib graft technique.

bilization is usually necessary until solid C-1/C-2 union has occurred. In addition, the transoral approach seems to have a greater chance of post-operative non-union and of course has an increased risk of postoperative sepsis. It should probably be considered only in the case of an anteriorly displaced, irreducible non-united fracture.

Problems of pure ligamentous injury without fracture at the atlanto-axial joint are less frequent but can be managed in a similar fashion when they demonstrate chronic instability (Fig. 9). These are rather unusual since most often the odontoid process fractures at its base before there is ligamentous disruption. Even more unusual are the occipito-atlantal subluxations (5,18,19) (Fig. 10). These injuries are often immediately fatal, but when associated with chronic instability they should be considered for a similar type of posterior fusion, which obviously should include the occiput (Fig. 11).

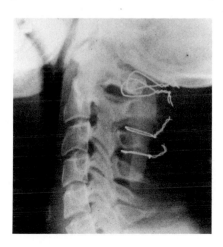

FIG. 8. Lateral view of C-1,2,3 fusion using the rib graft technique.

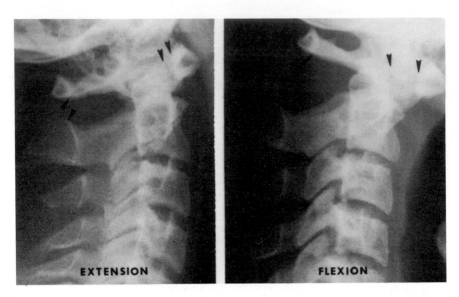

FIG. 9. Lateral flexion/extension views of the upper cervical spine demonstrating C-1/C-2 chronic instability due to ligamentous injury. In flexion, note the increased space between the odontoid process and the anterior C-1 arch.

As a matter of routine we have not included the occiput in the standard atlanto-axial fusion for C-1/C-2 instability, since it is not necessary for stabilization of the area with the rib graft technique and only further compromises motion in the upper cervical region.

Another situation of instability in the upper cervical area at the C-1/C-2 level is that occurring after upper respiratory infection. In general such problems occur in the pediatric age group and frequently the subluxation is

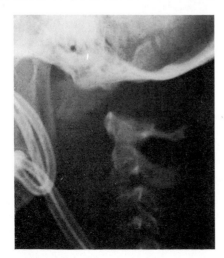

FIG. 10. Lateral view of the cervicocranial junction in a fatal case of atlanto-occipital subluxation.

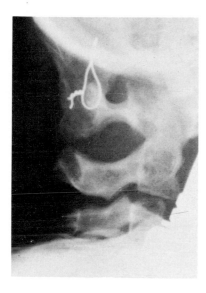

FIG. 11. Three months postoperative occipito-atlas fusion in a case of post-traumatic atlanto-occipital chronic instability.

unilateral, presenting as a "wry neck." In general they respond to traction and external immobilization, but under the circumstance of chronic instability one certainly should consider surgical fusion. With this situation the classic Gallie type of fusion between the C-1/C-2 laminae with iliac bone is probably more than adequate (4).

One additional and relatively common situation involving instability at the atlanto-axial joint is that associated with rheumatoid disease (2,12,13) (Fig. 12). As indicated previously, there is often a malformed or hypoplastic dens associated with this condition. With significant instability and related

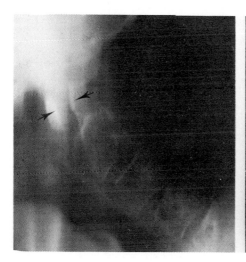
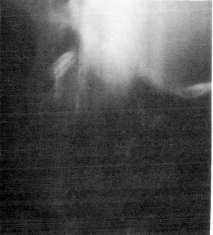

FIG. 12. Lateral flexion/extension view of the upper cervical spine demonstrating chronic C-1/C-2 instability in a case of rheumatoid arthritis.

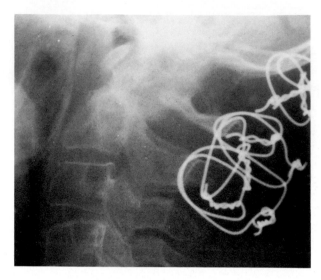

FIG. 13. Occipital-upper cervical fusion utilizing wires incorporated into acrylic struts.

symptomatology, and most particularly when associated with definite neurologic signs, posterior surgical fusion is certainly indicated. Under these circumstances and because of a greater postsurgical complication rate in these older patients, we attempt to expedite the surgical procedure as much as possible and often use wires incorporated into acrylic struts for support of the area (Fig. 13).

Similarly, developmental abnormalities in the upper cervical area (e.g., the os odontoideum) often have some degree of associated ligamentous instability (7) (Fig. 14). Most often these congenital abnormalities are isolated radiographic findings; but at times and especially when there is evident

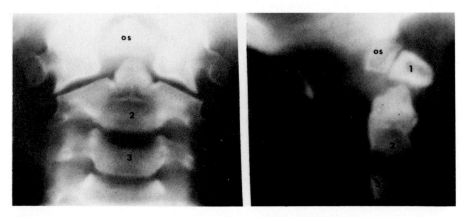

FIG. 14. Upper cervical tomograms demonstrating an os odontideum. These congenital abnormalities can be associated with chronic instability.

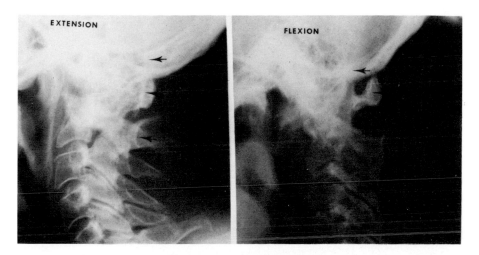

FIG. 15. Lateral views of the upper cervical area revealing occipito-atlanto-axial instability following transclival surgery for a basilar artery aneurysm.

instability, neurologic signs and symptoms can develop. When this is evident posterior fusion is recommended.

One final problem of some interest to the neurosurgeon is that of atlanto-axial instability following transclival surgery (Fig. 15). In this procedure removal of the anterior arch of C-1 and the odontoid process are usually a necessary part of the operation, and under these circumstances postoperative C-1/C-2 instability can evolve. If significant and symptomatic, one should consider these patients for posterior surgical fusion.

MID AND LOWER CERVICAL SPINE

Stable Spine with Progressive Deformity

Stable spinal conditions with deformity in the mid and lower cervical spine are most often traumatic in origin (Table 3). Classically posttraumatic vertebral collapse is described in association with a "teardrop" fracture (Fig. 16).

TABLE 3. *Mid and lower cervical spinal deformities*

Stable Spine with Progressive Deformity
    Posttraumatic "tear drop fracture"
    Neoplastic metastatic disease
    Postsurgical anterior fusion collapse
Spinal Instability with Deformity
    Posttraumatic
    Rheumatoid
    Postsurgical "wide" laminectomy
    Neurologic joint space denervation

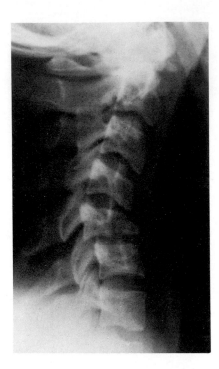

FIG. 16. Lateral cervical view demonstrating typical teardrop fracture of the fifth cervical vertebra.

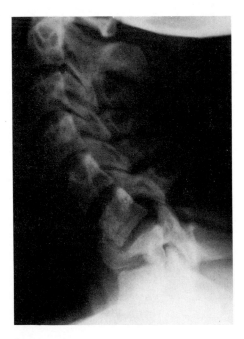

FIG. 17. Lateral cervical view some 4 months following injury in a case of an untreated teardrop fracture. Note the significant kyphosis that has developed.

Inadequate early support in these cases permits angulation to occur at the fracture site, and once the deformity has been allowed to develop it usually has a moderate degree of stability (Fig. 17). We favor approaching this problem anteriorly, with excision of the central portion of the deformed vertebral body back to the posterior longitudinal ligament and dura (9). This is relatively easy during the acute and subacute phases of healing, and correction of the spinal deformity is often accomplished without difficulty with the application of traction during the operative procedure (Fig. 18). In chronic cases where bony healing is more complete, correction of the deformity is often impossible, and one must be content with spinal cord decompression, without changing the overall vertebral deformity. We routinely use an iliac crest block graft to bridge the resultant vertebral body defect. Under most circumstances a postoperative period of external immobilization with a firm brace or halo vest is necessary until solid fusion occurs. Some surgeons advocate an acrylic strut to support and bridge the decompressed area. In general we do not consider this as a primary mode of treatment, but it could be an applicable alternative when it is necessary to excise a number of vertebral bodies. We attempt this acrylic technique only in cases where there is collapse due to multilevel tumor involvement requiring an extensive anterior decompression. This method requires fixation of the acrylic strut to adjacent solid bone with screws or wire (Fig. 19). These same general principles of management also apply to those cases of anterior cervical fusion in which there has been an unidentified early extrusion of the bone graft with secondary vertebral collapse and deformity.

Spinal Instability with Deformity

With regard to problems of ligamentous instability in the mid and lower cervical area, trauma again is the most frequent causative factor with subluxation through an intervertebral disc space or through a fracture site pseudoarthrosis (Fig. 20). Undoubtedly inadequate treatment plays a role in the initial development of these cases. We recommend reduction and realignment of the posttraumatic chronic subluxation followed by anterior fusion across the area of instability (Figs. 21 and 22). If the degree of instability is

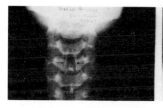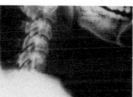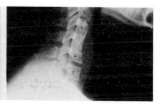

FIG. 18. Postoperative x-ray views of the case illustrated in Fig. 16, intermediate as well as some 20 months following surgery.

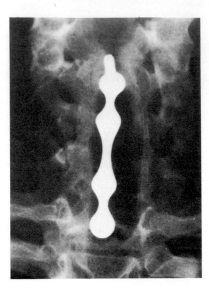

FIG. 19. Anteroposterior cervical x-ray in a case of extensive metastatic disease revealing a multilevel cervical fusion using an acrylic strut with additional support from a compression plate and screws embedded within the acrylic.

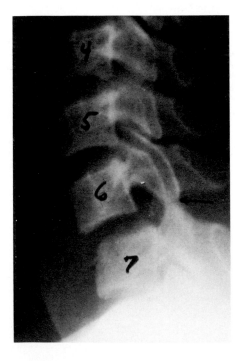

FIG. 20. Lateral cervical view revealing C-6/C-7 subluxation following an acute cervical injury.

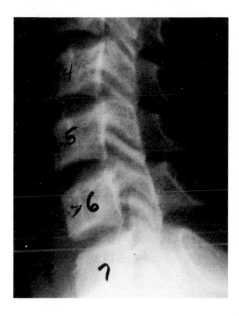

FIG. 21. Lateral cervical view of the case illustrated in Fig. 20 following traction and realignment of the subluxation.

large with significant ligamentous laxity, postoperative external immobilization is necessary since anterior fusion under these circumstances usually does not result in immediate solid stabilization of the area. As a very acceptable alternative, a posterior-type fusion could certainly be considered using iliac crest or rib struts and fusing, as a minimum, one adjacent lamina on either side of the involved levels.

Finally is the situation in the lower cervical spine in which there is an iatrogenic component, the "postlaminectomy" deformity (Fig. 23). Following an extensive laminectomy in some cases, a progressive angulation or "swan neck" deformity of the cervical spine can develop. At times it is quite

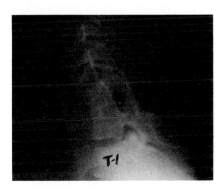

FIG. 22. Lateral cervical view of the case illustrated in Figs. 20 and 21 demonstrating stabilization of the C-6/C-7 level some 12 months following anterior fusion.

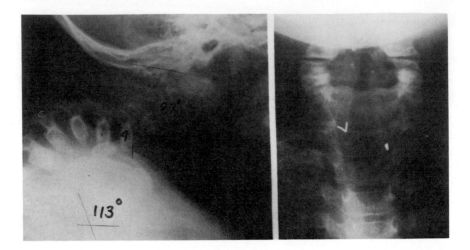

FIG. 23. Cervical x-ray views demonstrating a "swan neck" deformity several years following extensive laminectomy for an intramedullary spinal cord tumor in which the child had significant cervical sensory dysfunction.

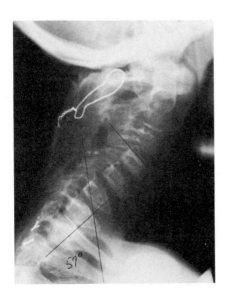

FIG. 24. Lateral cervical view of the case illustrated in Fig. 23 some months following partial traction reduction of the deformity and an extensive fusion involving the facets and lateral masses.

significant, and it seems to be particularly common in children following a procedure that involves multiple levels. Disruption of the facet joints compound the problem, and in a number of cases an additional factor is relevant, i.e., loss of joint space sensitivity due to primary pathology within the spinal cord, essentially then a problem of a "Charcot joint." An extensive laminectomy under the circumstances of significant joint sensory loss is almost certain to result in a troublesome postoperative spinal deformity. When confronted with this condition, attempted reduction of the deformity with traction is recommended followed by posterior fusion involving the facets and lateral masses (Fig. 24). Postoperative halo immobilization is necessary in these cases until solid fusion has occurred. Alternatively, one could consider a multilevel anterior fusion, but it does not seem to offer any significant advantage over the posterior approach. Not infrequently in the more severe deformities both methods need consideration.

SUMMARY

The spinal deformities of the cervical region should be considered under two broad categories. First are those problems that are related solely to bony collapse and angulation due to intrinsic osseus pathology. Management of these cases when the deformity is significant and especially when associated with neurologic impairment is that of decompression of the spinal cord with excision of the offending abnormality. This is usually carried out via an anterior cervical approach, which often creates or compounds any associated vertebral instability. As a consequence, then, in addition to the decompression, surgical stabilization is often necessary. In contrast, problems of spinal deformity related solely to instability are managed with a surgical stabilization procedure, either a posterior fusion (as in the case of the upper cervical spine) or anteriorly (which is usually the preferential method in the lower cervical area). With these principles of management, one can often successfully relieve spinal cord compression and its attendant neurologic symptoms.

REFERENCES

1. Braakman, R., and Penning, L. (1971): *Injuries of the Cervical Spine.* Excerpta Medica, Amsterdam.
2. Davidson, R. C., Ham, J. R., Herndon, J. H., and Grin, O. D. (1977): Brain stem compression in rheumatoid arthritis. *JAMA,* 238:2633–2634.
3. Fang, H. S. Y., and Ong, G. B. (1962): Direct or anterior approach to the upper cervical spine. *J. Bone Joint Surg.,* 44A:1588–1604.
4. Fielding, J. W., Hawkins, R. J., and Ratzan, S. A. (1976): Spine fusion for atlanto-axial instability. *J. Bone Joint Surg.,* 58A:400–407.
5. Gabrielsen, T. O., and Maxwell, J. A. (1966): Traumatic atlanto-occipital dislocation. *Am. J. Roentgenol. Radium Ther. Nucl. Med.,* 97:624–629.
6. Greenberg, A. D., Scoville, W. B., and Davey, L. M. (1968): Transnasal decompression of atlanto-axial dislocation. *J. Neurosurg.,* 28:266–269.

7. Hawkins, R. J., Fielding, W. J., and Thompson, W. J. (1976): Os-odontoideum: Congenital or acquired. *J. Bone Joint Surg.,* 58A:413–414.
8. Hensinger, R. N., and MacEwen, G. D. (1975): Congenital anomalies of the spine. In: *The Spine,* edited by R. H. Rothman and F. A. Simeone. Saunders, Philadelphia.
9. Johnson, R. M., and Southwick, W. O. (1975): Surgical approaches to the spine. In: *The Spine,* edited by R. J. Rothman and F. A. Simeone. Saunders, Philadelphia.
10. Kelly, D. L., Alexander, E., Davis, C. H., and Smith, J. M. (1972): Acrylic fixation of atlanto-axial dislocation. *J. Neurosurg.,* 36:366–371.
11. List, C. F. (1941): Neurologic syndromes accompanying developmental anomalies of occipital bone, atlas, and axis. *Arch. Neurol. Psychiatry,* 45:577–616.
12. Mathews, J. A. (1974): Atlanto-axial subluxation in rheumatoid arthritis. *Ann. Rheum. Dis.,* 33:526–531.
13. Mayer, J. W., Messner, R. P., and Kaplan, R. J. (1976): Brain stem compression in rheumatoid arthritis. *JAMA,* 236:2094–2095.
14. McGregor, M. (1948): The significance of certain measurements of the skull in the diagnosis of basilar impression. *Br. J. Radiol.,* 21:171–181.
15. McLauren, R. L., Vernal, R., and Salmon, J. H. (1972): Treatment of fractures of the atlas and axis by wiring without fusion. *J. Neurosurg.,* 36:773–780.
16. McRae, D. L. (1960): The significance of abnormalities of the cervical spine. *Am. J. Roentgenol. Radium Ther. Nucl. Med.,* 84:3–25.
17. Norrell, H. A. (1975): Fractures of the atlas and axis. In: *The Spine,* edited by R. H. Rothman and F. A. Simeone. Saunders, Philadelphia.
18. Page, C. P., Story, J. L., Wissinger, J. P., and Branch, C. L. (1973): Traumatic atlanto-occipital dislocation. *J. Neurosurg.,* 39:394–397.
19. Rockswold, G., and Seljeskog, E. L. (1978): Traumatic atlanto-occipital dislocation. *Minn. Med.,* 61:519–522.
20. Penning, L. (1968): *Functional Pathology of the Cervical Spine.* Williams & Wilkins, Baltimore.
21. Schneider, R. C., Livingston, K. E., Cave, A. J. E., and Hamilton, G. (1956): "Hangmans fracture" of the cervical spine. *J. Neurosurg.,* 22:141–154.
22. Scoville, W. B. (1951): Platybasia: Report of ten cases. *Ann. Surg.,* 133:496–502.
23. Seljeskog, E. L. (1978): Non-operative management of acute upper cervical injuries. *Acta Neurochirg.* 41: (*in press*).
24. Seljeskog, E. L., and Chou, S. N. (1978): Experiences and treatment of the odontoid fracture. *J. Neurosurg.* (*in press*).
25. Seljeskog, E. L., and Chou, S. N. (1976): The spectrum of the hangmans fracture. *J. Neurosurg.,* 45:3–8.
26. Southwick, W. O., and Robinson, R. A. (1957): Surgical approaches to the vertebral bodies. *J. Bone Joint Surg.,* 39A:631–644.
27. Spillane, J. D., Pallis, C., and Jones, A. M. (1957): Developmental abnormalities in the region of the foramen magnum. *Brain,* 80:11–48.
28. Sukoff, M. H., Koltin, M. M., and Moran, T. (1972): Transoral decompression for myelopathy caused by rheumatoid arthritis. *J. Neurosurg.,* 37:493–497.

Spinal Deformities and Neurological Dysfunction, edited by S. N. Chou and E. L. Seljeskog. Raven Press, New York © 1978.

Treatment of Thoracic Spinal Deformity with Neurological Deficit

Shelley N. Chou

Department of Neurosurgery, University of Minnesota Medical School, Minneapolis, Minnesota 55455

With the exception of trauma, neurological dysfunction associated with spinal deformity of the thoracic level is usually insidious in onset and slow in progression. The majority of such cases is associated with idiopathic or congenital spinal deformities, particularly kyphosis. Rarely tuberculous infection is the cause.

When a progressive neurological dysfunction is definitely established, the treatment in most cases is surgical decompression by an anterior approach. The classic laminectomy has no place here as it does not accomplish the purpose. Indeed it is contraindicated because it usually worsens the neurological deficit (6).

There are basically two surgical procedures that can be employed to decompress the spinal cord in the thoracic or thoracolumbar area under such conditions. They are the lateral rachotomy of Capener (1) or the transthoracic or transthoracic-retroperitoneal procedure popularized by Hodgson (5).

Before surgery is undertaken, the etiology of the spinal deformity should be ascertained. If it is a kyphosis, whether the apex is rigid or flexible must be determined by obtaining dynamic views on x-ray film, as a flexible apex sometimes can be reduced by judicious traction. Should the deformity be gradually and adequately reduced concomitant with neurological recovery, a posterior fusion may then be done. It is in such situations that the orthopedic and neurosurgical teams must work very closely to assess and adopt the best therapeutic approach.

A complete work-up for a surgical candidate should include the following steps:

a. Neurological examination—motor function, reflex changes, evidence of muscle fasciculation, and/or atrophy. Sensory examination for all modalities. Rectal examination for sphincter tone and sensation.

b. Roentgenological examination—x-ray study including tomography of the spine in a variety of views is important. The apical region of a kyphosis and/or scoliosis should be carefully studied as to its rigidity and degree of angulation. Associated deformities such as diastematomyelia may be seen.

c. Myelographic examination—large-volume contrast study is a must (4). Such a technique is mandatory to reveal the relationship of the skeletal and neural elements in the critical area of deformity; occasionally it shows occult, associated intraspinal lesions, e.g., a lipoma or diastematomyelia.

d. Neurourological study—using electronic means to evaluate the functions of the bladder, the vesical, and rectal sphincters. This involves a series of very sensitive urodynamic studies which are essential to understanding the total function of the spinal cord and the cauda equina with respect to the bladder function. Such studies are discussed elsewhere in this book.

Once the patient is fully worked up and the decision made that an anterior decompression is the procedure of choice, the question of whether to use the Capener or the Hodgson procedure should then be addressed. The *Capener procedure* is a retropleural approach and is useful for deformity of limited vertebral segments, usually less than two, and less angulation of much less than 90° (Fig. 1B). To perform such a procedure, the patient is placed in a prone position with appropriate support to decrease the intra-thoracic and intraabdominal pressure (Fig. 1A). A paramedian incision is employed and the paraspinal muscles are split down to the costotransverse junction. One or two ribs are exposed and their resections along with the transverse process are made to assure adequate exposure of the lateral aspect of the spinal column (Fig. 1A,C). The neurovascular bundle is followed into the intervertebral foramen. The pedicle is located and resected, and thus the spinal canal entered (Fig. 1D). When necessary the spinal nerve can be cut and the proximal segment gently elevated to expose the anterior aspect of the spinal canal. If further exposure is necessary, a limited laminectomy can be added to this procedure; more than 180° of the anterolateral spinal canal can be exposed in this way without excessive traction of the spinal cord. The kyphotic bone compressing the spinal cord can then be removed by subcortical curettage, and the cortical layer can be fractured with force directed away from the dural sac. The osteotectomy should start laterally, moving cautiously medially across the midline until satisfactory decompression is accomplished (Fig. 1E,F). Whether a fusion is necessary depends on a number of factors to be determined by the orthopedic team. Postoperative care in such cases is less complicated because the pleural cavity is not entered and no chest drainage is necessary.

For the *Hodgson procedure,* which is valuable for a severe kyphotic and/or scoliotic lesion, coordinated thoracic, neurosurgical, and orthopedic teamwork is necessary. It is best to study jointly the patient, the x-rays, and other important information (e.g., pulmonary function) in order to formulate the surgical plan.

As far as the preoperative care is concerned, the main function here is the assessment of pulmonary function. Some kyphotic and/or scoliotic patients have associated chest deformities which render the normal chest excursion impossible; the pulmonary function may be so poor that it makes

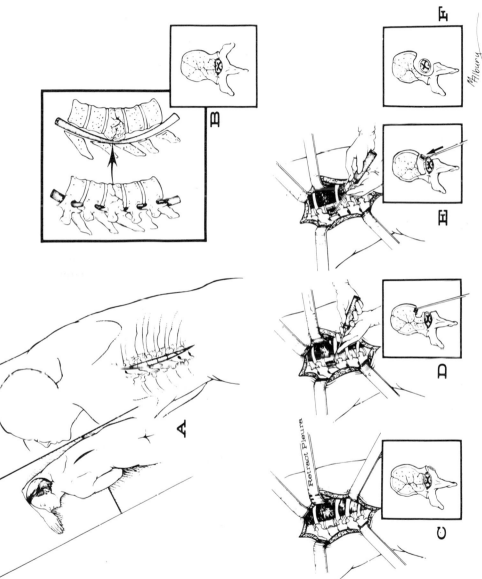

FIG. 1. Steps in a modified Capener procedure. See text for details.

this procedure far too risky for such a patient. It is important that anesthesiology consultations be obtained in advance; many patients must undergo a prolonged period of intensive pulmonary care prior to surgery.

For the intraoperative management the patient is placed in the decubitus position close to the edge of the operating table with the body well secured and the pressure points protected (Fig. 2A). During the procedure it may be necessary to rotate the operating table sideways to facilitate visualization into the spinal canal. A headlight is very useful for the surgeon because the usual operating room lighting is not adequate.

A right thoracotomy is used for a kyphotic patient. For patients with kyphoscoliosis the approach should be on the side of the concavity of the curve. Using this approach decompression of the spinal cord is anteriorly and at the pedicular compressive site as well. The thoracotomy incision (Fig. 1A) should be such that maximal exposure of the vertebral segments involved can be accomplished. Most of the time one rib is resected, but occasionally two ribs may have to be removed. These ribs are saved for anterior strut fusion by the orthopedic team after the decompression is accomplished. The ribs resected should be one or two segments above the kyphotic apex. The transverse process should be resected down to the vertebral body. A thoracotomy as described can bring as many as seven or eight vertebral segments into view. If the thoracolumbar area is involved, the diaphragm must be detached and the retroperitoneal space entered.

When the apex of the vertebral level is exposed (Fig. 2B) the pleura should be reflected and the osteotectomy begun at the area of the vertebral pedicular junction. First a gouge is used to remove the cancellous bone (Fig. 2C). When a sufficient canal is created, a large rongeur is used (Fig. 2D) to enlarge and lengthen the ostectomy. Gradually the canal is enlarged so that the posterior cortical bone surface is exposed. Then, using curved curettes, the cortical bone is gradually thinned and fractured piecemeal (Fig. 2E,F). It is important not to fracture the cortical bone in large pieces because it may snap back against the spinal cord. When the canal is created, the spinal cord elements gradually move into it (Fig. 2G).

During the bone removal there is usually significant oozing of blood from the vertebral bodies, so that long and large suction apparatus in pairs are necessary to keep the operative field clean. Sometimes it is a matter of continuing the osteotectomy with a curet by "feel" only because of the wet field, which is deep and obscured by blood.

The most difficult areas from which to remove the cortical bones are those close to the intervertebral discs. There is usually firm adhesions and thickening of the soft tissue thereabout.

After the bone is removed, the posterior longitudinal ligaments may or may not be an obvious structure that come into view next. When the ligament is thick, however, it should be incised longitudinally with a 12-bladed knife, which cuts from within, out. The leaves of the ligament should

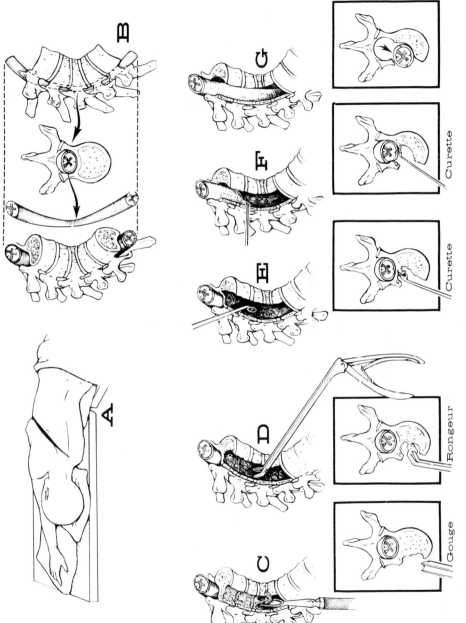

FIG. 2. Steps in a Hodgson procedure. See text for details.

be gently peeled off the dura and excised. This maneuver releases the epidural veins, which begin to bleed at this point, sometimes necessitating packing with Gelfoam or other hemostatic agents. Bipolar coagulation can be useful to control bleeding, but unipolar coagulation should be avoided because the heat generated may damage the spinal cord.

When adequate osteotectomy is accomplished and the longitudinal ligament excised, the dural sac gradually moves into the surgically created canal (Fig. 2G). Thus the caudad and cephalad ends of the bony canal may appear again to be compressing against the spinal cord. The osteotectomy should be extended both up and down to make sure adequate decompression has been accomplished.

The blood loss during surgery is fairly substantial, and it should be replaced by careful monitoring with a central venous pressure line or, more preferably, a Swan-Ganz catheter. Bleeding from the operative site should be controlled by packing with hemostatic agents such as Gelfoam. The orthopedic team takes over the operation at this point to do the strut fusion, and the thoracotomy is closed by the thoracic team. In the early stages of our experience we required 8–9 hr to perform such a procedure. At the present time it takes approximately 5 hr.

During the postoperative period the chest tubes for continuous drainage are cared for by the thoracic surgeons. Controlled respiration should be used initially with frequent blood gas determinations. Chest x-rays are taken to detect atelectasis, pneumonitis, and pleural fusions. These patients should be put on prophylactic antibiotics for a period of a week. If no significant complications take place these patients can be up with chest tubes removed in approximately a week. A plaster cast from the sternum to the pelvis is applied and usually stays for at least 3 months. Patients should receive physical therapy and gait training as soon as possible. Whether a posterior fusion procedure is subsequently necessary depends on the solidarity of the anterior fusion and the nature of the deformity of the spine.

It is important to check these patients neurologically during the long follow-up period, and appropriate x-ray assessment should also be made.

Our results with the transthoracic decompression and fusion have been excellent (2,3). We now have 35 consecutive cases with only three deaths. The three mortalities occurred early in our experience. We have had no mortality or postoperative neurological deterioration during the past 6 years.

SUMMARY

The surgical management of patients with thoracic spinal deformity and neurological dysfunction by either the Capener or the Hodgson procedure was described. The preoperative assessment, intraoperative technique, and postoperative follow-up are outlined. The importance of a multi-disciplinary approach to such problems is emphasized.

REFERENCES

1. Capener, N. (1954): The evolution of lateral rhacotomy. *J. Bone Joint Surg.*, 36B:173–179.
2. Chou, S. N. (1977): The treatment of paralysis with kyphosis. *Clin. Orthop.*, 128:149–154.
3. Chou, S. N., and Seljeskog, E. L. (1973): Alternative surgical approaches to the thoracic spine. *Clin. Neurosurg.*, 20:306–321.
4. Gold, L. H. A., Leach, D. G., Kieffer, S. A., Chou, S. N., and Peterson, H. O. (1970): Large volume myelography: An aid in the evaluation of curvature of the spine. *Radiology*, 97:531–636.
5. Hodgson, A. R., and Stock, F. E. (1956): Anterior spinal fusion: A preliminary communica-cation on the radical treatment of Pott's paraplegia. *Br. J. Surg.*, 44:266–275.
6. Lonstein, J. E., Winter, R. B., Moe, J. H., Bradford, D. S., Chou, S. N., and Pinto, M. C. (1978): Neurological deficits secondary to spinal deformity. *J. Bone Joint Surg.* (*in press*).

Spinal Deformities and Neurological Dysfunction, edited by S. N. Chou and E. L. Seljeskog. Raven Press, New York © 1978.

Treatment of Thoracolumbar Fractures with Associated Neurological Injury

Donald L. Erickson

Department of Neurological Surgery, University of Minnesota Hospital, Minneapolis, Minnesota 55455; and Department of Neurological Surgery, St. Paul Ramsey Hospital, St. Paul, Minnesota 55101

Spine trauma at the thoracolumbar junction requires special consideration owing to some unique problems related to that area. Firstly, the neurological trauma affects both spinal cord and cauda equina, which are tissues with vastly different potentials for recovery. Secondly, there is perhaps a greater potential for instability and late deformity due to the rigid thoracic spine above and the heavy load applied at that junction. Lack of attention to either of these aspects reduces the likelihood of adequate treatment. Incomplete decompression does not allow maximum neurological recovery. Poor stabilization may give rise to late deformity and recurrent neurological dysfunction.

The neurosurgeon's primary concern is to ensure adequate decompression in order to optimize the potential recovery. Although decompression has not generally been of value in spinal cord trauma, it is recommended for cauda equina injury (10,12,20). Laminectomy, a common form of spinal canal decompression, may add to instability and at times may deal inadequately with the deformity (4,5,10,12,13,20). Most of the fractures at this area are due to hyperflexion, producing either a dislocation or burst-type fracture. Laminectomy does not reduce the dislocation, nor does it allow easy removal of the burst vertebral body, which projects into the spinal canal (Fig. 1).

An alternate approach has been suggested in the form of anterior decompression and fusion (23). This does provide adequate decompression and ultimately produces a solid, stable spine; but it does not give immediate stability, and if one allows early mobilization there is a risk of slippage.

We propose a third alternative, which provides immediate stability and adequate decompression. This has become our standard approach for most thoracolumbar fracture over the past several years.

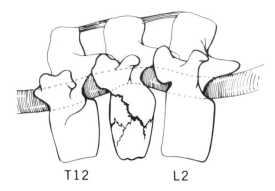

FIG. 1. Burst fracture with impingement on anterior aspect of spinal canal.

PATIENT SELECTION AND SURGICAL TECHNIQUE

The first five patients were seen between March and December 1973 and had either T12,L1 burst fractures or fracture-dislocations. Their neurological deficits were similar, each having saddle anesthesia, bladder and bowel paralysis, and varying degrees of lower extremity paresis and sensory loss. This neurological deficit, combined with evidence of compression of neural structures, was the indication for surgery. Myelography was not done routinely if the spine malalignment was of a degree sufficient to imply neural impingement but if there was reason to question the presence of of neural compression, myelography was used to elucidate it. In some patients, plane x-rays or laminograms were sufficient to determine this. If there was evidence of spinal cord and cauda equina compression, the patient was operated on when his general condition was stable. Emergency decompression is believed not warranted unless there is evidence of neurological deterioration. The benefit provided by surgery in patients with a stable neurological deficit is probably related to recovery of the cauda equina, rather than conus.

At surgery the patient is positioned on a four-point Hall frame, preventing any compression of the abdomen and also allowing some hyperextension to develop during surgery, which aids in reduction of the spinal deformity. A midline incision is made sufficiently long to expose five vertebral segments, which is necessary for insertion of the Harrington rods. The muscle is reflected bilaterally and the posterior elements examined. If the posterolateral elements on one side appear to be less stable, that side is chosen to initiate the decompression. On rare occasions one finds severe disruption of the lamina and dura, with cauda equina entangled in bone fragments (8). In that situation, any initial attempt at stabilization is abandoned and all efforts are directed toward obtaining adequate decompression and approximating the tissue layers. The more typical situation is to find a relatively

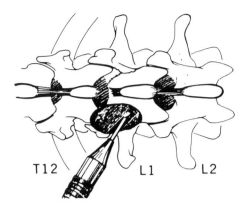

FIG. 2. Removal of lateral lamina and pedicle.

intact canal, in which event the muscle is then reflected more widely on the chosen side until the entire facet joint at the site of the fracture is exposed. Using rongeur and air drill (Fig. 2) the lateral lamina, facet, and pedicle are removed at the level which allows lateral exposure of the area of spinal deformity. The exiting nerve root is identified and the lateral dural sac well exposed at the area of the fracture, similar to a costotranversectomy approach. If there are any obvious loose bone or disc fragments within the canal, they are removed initially. More often, however, the anterior deformity is due to the retropulsed comminuted burst fracture of the L1 vertebral body. This is dealt with by entering directly into the vertebral body, lateral to the dural sac, and undermining the body beneath the sac, leaving only a thin shell of cortical bone (Fig. 3). It is important to leave this posterior cortex until sufficient vertebral body has been removed because it offers protection for the overlying neural elements during the cureting process. Once this has been thoroughly undermined, the thin cortical shell can be fractured anteriorly away from the dural sac, accomplishing the

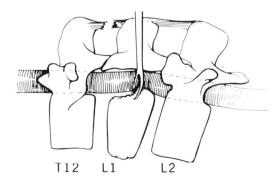

FIG. 3. Curettement of vertebral body.

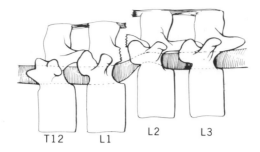

FIG. 4. Fracture dislocation.

decompression without need for retraction of the dura (19). The dural sac migrates anteriorly, and dural pulsations return distal to the area of compression. One can confirm the adequacy of decompression by passing a curved dissector beneath the dural sac to the opposite side of the spinal canal. Hemostasis can be readily achieved with gel-foam pledgets and bone wax.

With decompression of neural elements accomplished, the second phase — stabilization — commences. The details of Harrington rod insertion are discussed in another section and elsewhere (2,6,7). The decompression exposure allows one to observe the effects of the rod distraction and be assured that no damage to neural elements occurs.

If one finds, after exposure of the anterior lateral aspect of the canal, that the compression is due strictly to dislocation, it is unnecessary to remove the vertebral body as described above. As realignment is restored with the application of Harrington rods, observable decompression is accomplished as well (Figs. 3, 4 and 5). Even with pure dislocations it is not unusual to see disc fragments within the canal; these should be removed prior to insertion of the Harrington rods. Following surgery, the patient can be moved directly to a standard hospital bed. Postoperative care is simplified in that the patient can be moved readily from side to side without fear of spinal instability. Within 1 to 2 weeks, a body cast or appropriate brace is applied, and the

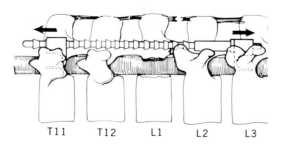

FIG. 5. Realignment with Harrington rods.

patient begins sitting or standing, depending on the degree of neurological deficit. Active rehabilitation on the physical medicine and rehabilitation services is then begun. A well-padded, bivalved cast that can be removed when the patient is recumbent is recommended to enhance skin care.

RESULTS

These five patients were operated between March and December 1973 and have been followed in the outpatient department with serial x-rays and neurological examinations. Results can be assessed in three categories: (a) duration of hospitalization; (b) stability of the spine; and (c) neurological function.

The average hospital stay was 77 days, which compares favorably with that reported for similar injuries in other studies (2,6,16,24). This can be attributed in part to the early stability, allowing mobilization within 1–2 weeks of the injury. Also important is the patient's motivation, which is much enhanced if he is active and progressing, rather than bedfast during the inevitable period of postinjury depression.

All five of these patients developed stable spines that required no further surgical intervention and that had no progression of deformity (14,15,21). Back pain, which is a common complaint when stabilization is not done, was present in none of these patients (12,18).

Neurologically, there was no deterioration associated with the surgical procedure (19). All five patients had neurological improvement over the subsequent year, at least, indicating that decompression was adequate. They are all walking; one requires no bracing, and the others ambulate with short leg braces. One had ileal diversion, and another uses a condom catheter. The other three are catheter-free, in spite of the fact that all have persistent saddle anesthesia or marked hypesthesia.

DISCUSSION

Comprehensive treatment of thoracolumbar fracture with attendant neurological injury requires not only decompression but attention to stability as well. Neurosurgeons have often ignored stability in an attempt at achieving adequate decompression. Orthopedic surgeons have at times been so concerned with stabilization that decompression has taken second place (3,4,14,17).

If stabilization is inadequate, late-onset deformity can occur and increase neurological deficits (21,22). If decompression is not optimal, potentially salvageable cauda equina may not recover. Only when the surgeon has accomplished both goals has he provided the best care for his patient.

Most thoracolumbar fractures have an anterior defect due to vertebral body burst or dislocation step-off, and simply removing the lamina does not deal adequately with the anterior aspect of the deformity. Unless one deals with the anterior, as well as the posterior, aspect of the deformity, the decompression is often unsatisfactory. Attempts at removing the anterior offending defect via a standard laminectomy are often difficult and may require excessive retraction of the dural sac and spinal cord (19). Also, to achieve significant decompression with laminectomy, at least three lamina should be removed, which can result in increased instability and make subsequent stabilizing attempts more difficult. The large posterior defect that is a necessary part of decompressive laminectomy carries a risk of subsequent epidural hematoma; and in patients with marked neurological deficit, postoperative assessment of this complication is difficult. A decompressive laminectomy without subsequent stabilization requires a prolonged period of bed rest which is undesirable physiologically and psychologically. The anterior retroperitoneal approach likewise does not produce immediate stability and it also would not be as useful for pure dislocations (9,13,19). Several other methods of prosthetic stabilization have been advocated, but they do not provide simultaneous decompression (1,2,5,10,12).

We therefore suggest that the ideal treatment of these injuries is decompression of the neural elements, restoration of the spinal alignment, and immediate stabilization, with a minimal exposure of the spinal canal. The one-stage decompression stabilization procedure described in this section is our attempt to achieve this. The anterior aspect of the defect is readily dealt with through the posterior lateral approach, and the realignment and stabilization is accomplished with insertion of Harrington rods. This decompression produces little instability, and the Harrington rods readily resolve even that, making early mobilization and rehabilitation conceivable (2,6,7,11). The relatively small exposure of the dural sac makes the complication of epidural hematoma less likely. We have seen no increase in neurological deficit related to this approach, and we shortened the average hospital stay for these patients by at least 3 to 4 weeks. Even though definite improvement in neurological function has been observed following this procedure, we are reluctant to say that it would not also have occurred with other forms of treatment or spontaneously. It must be recognized, however, that laminectomy alone may not fully decompress the cauda equina if it is tethered over an anterior deformity (21,22).

The pattern of neurological loss most commonly seen initially is saddle anesthesia, bladder and bowel paralysis, and varying degrees of lower-extremity paresis and sensory loss. Neurological recovery generally occurs only in the lower extremities, suggesting recovery of the cauda equina but not of the conus (10). The value of decompression of nerves that have a reasonable potential for recovery is emphasized (10,12,20).

It is our conviction that the cooperation of orthopedic and neurological surgeons, allowing the coordination of the two operative procedures, has been beneficial to our patients. We have therefore continued to use this approach during the past 4 years with similar results.

SUMMARY

(a) A one-stage decompression stabilization procedure for thoracolumbar fractures is described.

(b) Results suggest that it is a safe and effective procedure to deal with this problem.

(c) The procedure significantly shortens the period of hospitalization without compromising the clinical recovery.

(d) A more adequate decompression than with laminectomy alone is obtained, and the decompression is better maintained.

REFERENCES

1. Bohler, J. L. (1970): Operative treatment of fractures of the dorsal and lumbar spine. *J. Trauma*, 10:1119–1122.
2. Dickson, J. H., Harrington, P. R., and Erwin, W. D. (1973): Harrington instrumentation in the fractured, unstable thoracic and lumbar spine. *Texas Med.*, 69:91–98.
3. Frankel, H. L., Hancock, D. O., Hyslop, G., Melzak, J., Michaelis, L. S., Ungar, G. H., Vernon, J. D., and Walsh, J. J. (1969): The value of postural reduction in the initial management of close injuries of the spine with paraplegia and tetraplegia. *Paraplegia*, 7:179–192.
4. Guttman, L. (1969): Spinal deformities in traumatic paraplegics and tetraplegics following surgical procedures. *Paraplegia*, 7:38–58.
5. Hardy, A. G. (1965): The treatment of paraplegia due to fracture-dislocations of the dorso-lumbar spine. *Paraplegia*, 3:112–119.
6. Harrington, P. R. (1967): Technical details in relation to the successful use of instrumentation in scoliosis. *Orthop. Clin. North Am.*, 3.49–67.
7. Harrington, P. R. (1972): Instrumentation in spine instability other than scoliosis. *South Afr. J. Surg.*, 5:7–12.
8. Harris, P. (1968): Organization of spinal units. *Paraplegia*, 5:133–137.
9. Hodgson, A. R., Stock, F. E., Fane, H. S. Y., and Ong, G. B. (1960): Anterior spinal fusion, the operative approach and pathological findings in 412 patients with Pott's disease of the spine. *Br. J. Surg.*, 48:172–178.
10. Holdsworth, F. (1963): Fractures, dislocations, and fracture-dislocations of the spine. *J. Bone Joint Surg.*, 45B:6–20.
11. Katznelson, A. M. (1969): Stabilization of the spine in traumatic paraplegia. *Paraplegia*, 7:33–37.
12. Kaufer, H., and Hayes, J. T. (1966): Lumbar fracture-dislocation. *J. Bone Joint Surg.*, 48A:712–730.
13. Kelly, R. P., and Whitesides, T. E. (1968): The treatment of lumbo-dorsal fracture dislocation. *Ann. Surg.*, 167:705–717.
14. Leidholdt, J. D., Young, J. J., Hahn, H. R., Jackson, R. E., Gamble, W. E., and Miles, J. S. (1969): Evaluation of the late spinal deformities with fracture-dislocations of the dorsal and lumbar spine in paraplegics. *Paraplegia*, 7:16–27.
15. McSweeney, T. (1968): Spinal deformity after spinal cord injury. *Paraplegia*, 6:212–221.
16. Meyer, P. R. (1973): Annual Report, Midwest Regional Spinal Cord Injury Care System, Chicago.
17. Munro, D. (1965): The role of fusion or wiring in the treatment of acute traumatic instability of the spine. *Paraplegia*, 3:97 111.
18. Nicoll, E. A. (1949): Fractures of the dorso-lumbar spine. *J. Bone Joint Surg.*, 31B:376–394.

19. Norrell, H. (1975): Fractures and dislocations of the spine. In: *The Spine,* Vol. II, edited by R. H. Rotham and F. A. Simeone. Saunders, Philadelphia.
20. Ransohoff, J. (1970): Lesions of the cauda equina. *Clin. Neurosurg.,* 17:331–334.
21. Roberts, J. B., and Curtiss, P. H. (1970): Stability of the thoracic and lumbar spine in traumatic paraplegia following fracture or fracture-dislocation. *J. Bone Joint Surg.,* 52A: 1115–1130.
22. Schneider, R. C. (1962): Indications and contraindications in spine and spinal cord trauma. *Clin. Neurosurg.,* 8:157.
23. Whitesides, T. E., and Ghazanfar, A. S. (1976): On the management of unstable fractures of the thoracolumbar spine: rationale for use of anterior decompression and fusion and stabilization. *Spine,* 1:99.
24. Wilcox, N. E. Stauffer, E. S., and Nickel, V. L. (1970): A statistical analysis of 423 consecutive patients admitted to the spinal cord injury center, Rancho Los Amigos Hospital, 1 January 1964 through 31 December 1967. *Paraplegia,* 8:27–35.

Spinal Deformities and Neurological Dysfunction, edited by S. N. Chou and E. L. Seljeskog. Raven Press, New York © 1978.

Spine Fusion

Roby C. Thompson, Jr.

Department of Orthopedic Surgery, University of Minnesota Medical School, Minneapolis, Minnesota 55455

The biologic phenomenon involved in creating a fusion of one or more joints in the spine is essentially the study of fracture healing. When we approach a spine to create a fusion, we first establish fracture surfaces by denuding the bony elements of soft tissue and articular cartilage. Once the vascular cancellous surfaces have been established, they are then connected with a bone graft. In children, the periosteum is active in new bone formation, and simply stripping the periosteum and bridging the joint with bone grafts appears to be adequate for fusion of the cervical spine. The opposite situation is true in adult lumbar fusions; here meticulous technique is indicated to provide good apposition of cancellous bony surfaces between bone grafts and vertebral elements in order to achieve an acceptable rate of success.

Autografts of cancellous, corticocancellous, or cortical bone have distinct characteristics. *Cancellous bone* has the advantage of providing viable osteoblastic cells if the bone is handled properly. Surface cells in autogenous cancellous bone survive for a distance of approximately 1 mm from plasmatic circulation (10). Thus the ideal cancellous bone graft would be a strip of bone 2 mm at its thickest portion, providing viable osteocytes and osteoblasts on the surface of that graft with the matrix functioning as an architectural bridgework for new bone formation. Autogeneic cancellous bone establishes its new vascular supply by microanastomoses, which support proliferation of osteoprogenitor cells in a matter of a few days (10).

Cortical bone grafts are useful in providing internal fixation and for bridging large defects, e.g., vertebral body excision. Few if any surface cells survive in a cortical bone graft. However, if the graft is well handled, the ends of the graft are rapidly incorporated into the recipient surfaces and the graft is then revascularized and replaced with new bone. In large cortical grafts this "creeping substitution" may take as long as 13 years for replacement to occur. Combinations of cortical and cancellous bone [such as that used in the Smith-Robinson technique (8) for anterior interbody fusion] provide cancellous surfaces for early revascularization and osteogenesis while the cortical surfaces provide internal support. Allografts may also be useful in filling large defects in the spine since they function as architectural struts for new bone formation and may provide internal fixation for a transient period while there is new bone formation from supplemental autogeneous bone or periosteal new bone formation (10).

INTERNAL FIXATION VERSUS EXTERNAL FIXATION

As a supplement to the fracture healing discussed above, we normally utilize some sort of fixation device, either internal or external. Fractures of the spine treated by closed methods with external fixation rely on the intrinsic ability of the body to heal, either by spontaneous intervertebral fusion or by adequate soft tissue healing to provide support for the spinal column. Intervertebral element fusion for nontraumatic conditions also may require external or internal fixation devices. A good example of the need for internal fixation combined with external fixation is scoliosis fusions. In this type of fusion, not only are intervertebral elements healing to bone grafts, but major corrective forces have been applied to the spine. Thus the internal fixation devices used in scoliosis fusions not only hold the spine in a corrected position during the fusion process but also provide elements of immobilization to allow the fractures to heal. Because of the significant forces at play in this type of fusion, external fixation is also utilized in most instances. In those areas where large sheer forces are applied by virtue of the configuration of the spine (e.g., the occiput C1 and C1–C2 level), more rigid immobilization is required than at the midthoracic level where the rib cage provides additional intrinsic stability. Thus a fractured odontoid might be treated with a halo body cast, whereas a fracture in the midthoracic spine may be treated symptomatically or with a brace for comfort.

UPPER CERVICAL SPINE FUSION:
INDICATIONS AND TECHNIQUES

Occipitocervical fusion is indicated when there is occipitocervical instability. This most commonly is associated with assimilation of the atlas into the occiput or basilar invagination of the atlas into the occiput associated with a Klippel-Feil abnormality or other metabolic bone diseases as outlined by McRae in his treatise on upper cervical anomalies (3). Occipitocervical fusion is rarely indicated for instability between C1 and C2 alone, since the disability of an occipitocervical fusion is significantly greater than an atlantoaxial fusion (2). The technique of occipitocervical arthrodesis requires meticulous attention to detail with good autogenous cortical cancellous bone grafts supplemented with external fixation for a period of at least 12 weeks. The author prefers the use of a halo body cast for this procedure.

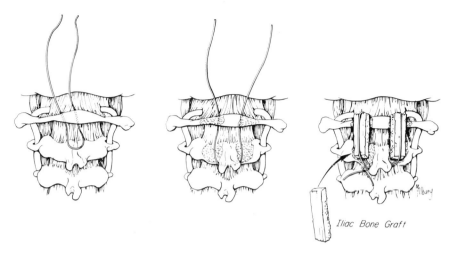

Iliac Bone Graft

FIG. 1. Modified Gallie fusion C1–C2 with corticocancellous strips wired between posterior elements of C1–C2. The wire loop was passed from cephalad to provide a better lever arm for correcting anterior displacement.

Atlantoaxial arthrodesis is most easily accomplished through the posterior approach. The technique as described by Gallie has been modified by several authors (4,8) but basically incorporates a loop of wire around the ring of C1 and the spinous process of C2 supplemented with corticocancellous bone grafts (Fig. 1). The author, again, in most circumstances prefers a halo body cast for external immobilization postfusion unless there is minimal instability present at the time of fusion.

Indications for atlantoaxial arthrodesis are based on instability of the C1–C2 complex either as a result of transverse ligament tears or fractures of the odontoid (1,4). Rheumatoid arthritis may produce instability requiring either atlantoaxial (6) or occipitocervical (7) arthrodesis (Fig. 2).

Posterior cervical spine fusions below the level of C2 are indicated for the management of locked facet joints and certain other traumatic conditions even though most surgeons prefer the anterior interbody approach when appropriate. Posterior fusions are also indicated in the management of neoplasia, etc. (8). The same fusion principles apply here; thus the author prefers a figure-eight type of wire to fix corticocancellous grafts in position (Fig. 3). This allows external immobilization to be reduced to a four-poster or sterno-occipito-mandibular-immobilizer (SOMI) type of brace. In the presence of extensive laminectomy, when anterior fusion is contraindicated or not possible, lateral interfacet joint fusions were popularized by Robinson and Southwick (9). These are technically difficult but feasible operations; they usually require the use of rib bone or fibular grafts for support combined with significant external immobilization such as a halo body cast (8).

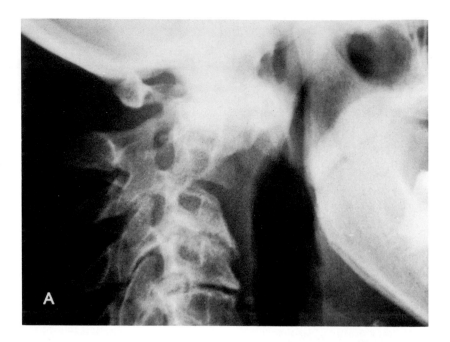

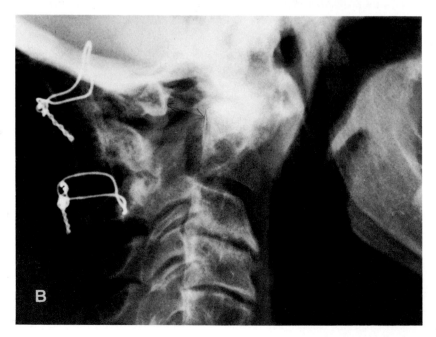

FIG. 2. A: Anterior subluxation of C1 on C2 in rheumatoid arthritis associated with occipitalization of the atlas. This situation requires occipital cervical fusion, as in **B.**

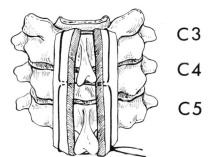

C3

C4

C5

FIG. 3. Figures-of-eight were passed through spinous process of C3, around corticocancellous grafts, and back through the interspinous space at C3–C4 to be secured beneath the spine of C5.

LUMBOSACRAL FUSION

Indications for lumbosacral fusion vary tremendously. The use of lumbosacral arthrodesis for low back pain in the author's experience is a much less common procedure today than it was 15 years ago. Based on personal experience I do not consider a herniated disc, "unstable" low back, or the presence of a congenital anomaly, *prima facie* indications for lumbar spine fusions. Painful and symptomatic spondylolisthesis as discussed by Bradford (*this volume*) is the least controversial area for lumbosacral spine fusion. However, lumbar spine fusion is occasionally indicated in patients with intractable back pain associated with definite osteoarthritis of the lumbar facet joints with or without congenital anomalies. The technique preferred by most orthopedic surgeons for lumbar spine fusion today employs the posterolateral fusion as the method of obtaining ankylosis between the lower lumbar vertebra and/or the sacrum (11,12). This procedure may be done through a midline incision in combination with laminectomy and/or nerve root decompression, or through separate lateral incision. Surgical technique in this area is critical, with meticulous attention to the detail of decortication, harvesting grafts, and application of the grafts to the spine. Using this technique, most surgeons agree there is no advantage to plaster cast immobilization or prolonged bed rest for the lumbosacral spine fusion, assuming that major structural defects are not being corrected at the same time the fusion is attempted.

Prothero and colleagues (5) compared 500 lumbar spine fusions done between 1959 and 1963 with 500 done between 1951 and 1953 at the same institution. During the first period of this study all patients were treated with prolonged bed rest, and during the second period they were ambulated within the first 3–4 days. No difference was noted in the fusion rate during these two decades. Other authors agree that early mobilization following lumbosacral spine fusion is advantageous since it allows rapid vascularization of the graft bed where autogenous corticocancellous bone is used.

METHYLMETHACRYLATE STABILIZATION FOR SPINE INSTABILITY

The use of a rapidly setting polymer such as methylmethacrylate for achieving stability of spine elements is theoretically attractive. However, mechanical studies have shown that methylmethacrylate is weak in shear; and with the tremendous shear forces applied through the spine, methylmethacrylate breaks loose from the bone with time. Thus short-term internal fixation of the spine with methylmethacrylate may be indicated in patients with instability and short life expectancy following metastatic disease to the spine, or in patients where spontaneous interbody fusion is anticipated and internal rather than external fixation is desired. There is no evidence to support the use of methylmethacrylate as a means of permanent fixation of vertebral elements in otherwise healthy individuals. The author reserves the use of methylmethacrylate for metastatic disease where significant intervertebral instability is present and life expectancy is shortened. Multiple interspinal wires are used as a core for the methacrylate, which is carefully interdigitated between the spinous processes, over the lamina, and around the previously positioned wire fixation (Fig. 4). Following this

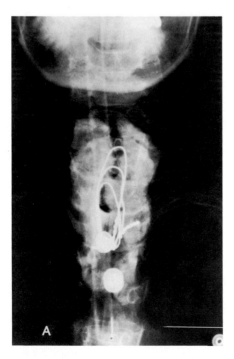 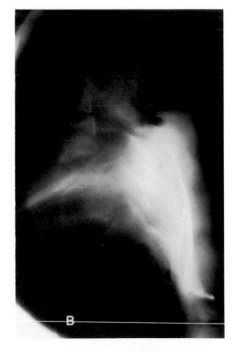

FIG. 4. Methylmethacrylate stabilization in pathologic fracture. Barium-filled methacrylate can be seen surrounding fixation wires that span the posterior elements where the entire body of T1 is destroyed by tumor.

technique, rapid mobilization of the patient is carried out with no external support other than a soft collar in the cervical spine or a brace in the lumbar spine.

REFERENCES

1. Fielding, J. W., Cochran, G. V. B., Lawsing, J. F., III, and Hohl, M. (1974): Tears of the transverse ligament of the atlas. *J. Bone Joint Surg.*, 56A:1683–1691.
2. Granthan, A. H., Dick, H. M., Thompson, R. C., and Stinchfield, F. E (1969): Occipito-cervical arthrodesis. *Clin. Orthop.*, 65:118–129.
3. MacRae, D. L. (1960): Significance of abnormalities of the cervical spine. *Am. J. Rheun-genol.*, 84:3.
4. McGraw, R. W., and Rusch, R. M. (1973): Atlanto-axial arthrodesis. *J. Bone Joint Surg.*, 55B:482–489.
5. Prothero, R. A., Parks, J. C., and Stinchfield, F. E. (1966): Complications after low back fusion in one thousand patients. *J. Bone Joint Surg.*, 48A:51–65.
6. Ranna, N. A., Hancock, D. O., Taylor, A. R., and Hill, A. G. S. (1973): Atlantosubluxa-tion in rheumatoid arthritis. *J. Bone Joint Surg.*, 55B:458–470.
7. Ranna, N. A., Hancock, D. O., Taylor, A. R., and Hill, A. G. S. (1973): Upper transloca-tion of the dens in rheumatoid arthritis. *J. Bone Joint Surg.*, 55B:471–477.
8. Robinson, R. A., and Riley, L. H. (1975): Techniques of exposure and fusion of the cervi-cal spine. *Clin. Orthop.*, 109:78–84.
9. Robinson, R. A., and Southwick, W. O. (1960): Indications and techniques for early stabi-lization of the neck in some fracture dislocations of the cervical spine. *South. Med. J.*, 53:568.
10. Urist, M. R. (1976): Practical application of basic research on bone graft psychology. In-structional Course Lecture, the American Academy of Orthopaedic Surgery, Vol. 25, pp. 1–26.
11. Watkins, M. B. (1964): Posterolateral fusion in pseudoarthrosis and posterior element defects of the lumbosacral spine. *Clin. Orthop.*, 35:80–85.
12. Wiltse, L. L., Bateman, G. J. G., Hutchison, R. H., and Nelson, W. E. (1968): The para-spinal sacrispinalous splitting approach to the lumbar spine. *J. Bone Joint Surg.*, 50A: 919–926.

*Spinal Deformities and Neurological
Dysfunction*, edited by S. N. Chou and
E. L. Seljeskog. Raven Press, New York
© 1978.

Role of Internal Fixation and Spine Fusion in Thoracic and Lumbar Spine Fractures

David S. Bradford

*Department of Orthopedic Surgery, University of Minnesota,
Minneapolis, Minnesota 55455*

Deformities of the axial skeleton following trauma have only recently begun to receive the attention they rightfully deserve. During the past decade, a greater awareness and appreciation of acute and chronic complications associated with spinal injuries have resulted in a more rational basis for early and long-term management. It is the purpose of this chapter to outline the indications and techniques of internal fixation in thoracic and lumbar spine injuries as it relates primarily to the neurological condition of the patient at the time of injury, as well as the status of bony and soft tissue stability of the vertebral column.

Although open reduction and fusion of a fracture dislocation of the spine was recommended by Albee in 1940 (1), most surgeons adopted nonoperative reduction of fracture dislocations by manipulation followed by immobilization in a plaster cast or plaster bed. During the second World War, Guttmann introduced the method of postural reduction (11). Primary consideration was given to prevention and management of neurologic complications while recognizing that the fracture of the spine, like any other, must be reduced and immobilized. By the skillful use of pillows and packs, the force of gravity facilitated reduction of the deformity and immobilization of the spine in the recumbent patient. Holdsworth and Hardy in 1953 revived open reduction (17), stating that neurologic recovery could best be facilitated by rapid restoration of normal spine alignment and stabilization of the fracture. They claimed that the stabilization with Williams plates made nursing care less difficult and improved the ultimate function of the spine and recovery of lumbar nerve roots. Pennypacker in 1953 (27) also suggested that this type of internal fixation would prevent progressive angulation of the spine. Dick (7) claimed that spines thus stabilized rendered ordinary nursing handling safe, preventing further damage to recovering nerve roots. Hardy in 1965 (14) found that there was no difference in neurologic results between nonoperative and operative cases in terms of neurologic recovery. Internal fixation for spine fractures received the greatest criticism from Guttmann in 1969 (13). He reviewed the records of over 100 patients in whom open reduction with metal plates had been carried out and concluded that the method did not prevent redislocation, regardless of the type of metal plate used, and that it was not unusual for plates to become loose and cut out of the spinous processes, and have to be removed. He also felt that the plates were detrimental and caused patients pain and increased rigidity of the spine. Furthermore, he stated that the patients did not obtain better neurologic recovery, and in fact there were instances of clinical deterioration following surgery.

A new method of internal fixation was advocated by Harrington et al. in 1960 (8) and later reports indicated that with this technique the rehabilitation, regardless of neurological recovery, was shortened as much as 400% (15,16). Reports by other authors since that time have confirmed that the technique is safe, improves nursing care, shortens rehabilitation, and is effective in maintaining fracture reduction and bony healing (3–5,8,9,18, 21,28).

More recently new techniques of internal fixation, consisting of Weiss springs, have been introduced. This method of internal fixation is also stated to decrease hospitalization time markedly and allow the patient more rapid mobilization without necessitating external support or even spine fusion. Although long-term experience has not been reported in the United States, the technique appears to be most useful when the posterior elements, including the facet joints, are still intact (6,25). Complications, however, appear to be considerable (more frequent than those associated with the Harrington device), and the final reduction and stabilization of the fracture appears to be inferior.

Recent work by Lewis and McKibben (24) compared two series of patients, one treated by open reduction and plating of unstable thoracolumbar spines and the other treated by postural reduction and nonoperative methods. Although no difference in neurological recovery could be detected between the two groups, the number treated conservatively had significant residual spinal deformity and subsequently developed serious pain that did not occur in any of the patients treated by plating.

INDICATIONS FOR OPEN REDUCTION AND INTERNAL FIXATION

In light of our own experience and that reported by Lewis and McKibben as well as Frankel et al. in 1969 (10), it is apparent that conservative measures often fail to reduce a displaced fracture of the thoracic and lumbar spine, especially if the displacement is greater than half the diameter of the vertebral body. The patients may be left with significant spine deformity and subsequent pain and disability. We believe that unstable fractures and stable fractures made unstable by decompression are best managed by open reduction, internal fixation, and spine fusion. The most important consideration, from the fracture standpoint, is the determination as to whether the injury is a stable or an unstable one and, if it is unstable, whether further displacement may be expected immediately or months to years after the injury. The work of Nicoll (26) and Holdsworth and Hardy (17) defined spine stability based on radiographic evaluation of the fracture. These authors noted that the stability of the vertebral column is dependent to a great degree on soft-tissue support. Posteriorly, the supraspinal and interspinal ligaments along with the capsules of the posterolateral joints and ligamentum flava produce what has become known as the "posterior ligament complex." The integrity of this complex is essential for spinal stability. Anteriorly, the intervertebral disc, the periosteum, and the anterior/posterior longitudinal ligaments provide additional functional support. One can consider the spine as two connecting columns—an anterior column consisting of vertebral bodies, disc, and ligaments; and a posterior column consisting of a neural arch, facet joints, and ligaments (Fig. 1).

Injuries to the spine may damage one or both of these columns and in the process produce varying degrees of spinal instability. It is important to determine whether the instability is acute or chronic. Acute instability implies a fracture that is capable of further displacement immediately after injury with resultant neurologic damage. Translational displacement anterior/posterior or medial/lateral as well as flexion/rotation (slice fracture of Holdsworth) result in acute instability, usually with neurologic deficit. Chronic instability implies an injury that may further angulate, producing greater deformity months or even years after injury. Therefore slow and

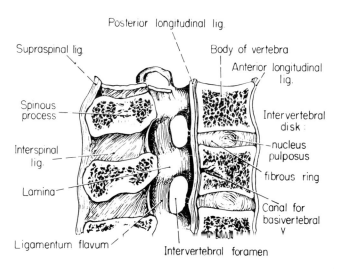

FIG. 1. Anatomy of the vertebral column may be considered as two structural columns: an anterior column consisting of vertebral bodies, discs, and ligaments; and a posterior column consisting of a neural arch, facet joints, and intervening ligaments. (From ref. 29.)

progressive neurological damage may result from chronic instability but only as a late consequence of marked angulation. Disruptions of both anterior and posterior columns or disruptions of the posterior ligament complex result in acute instability. Chronic instability is less common but may result from damage to the anterior column at one level (severe burst fractures) over multiple levels (multiple compression fractures) or following surgical procedures (i.e., laminectomy) which jeopardize the integrity of the posterior column.

The urgency and type of stabilization or instrumentation is dependent not only on the instability of the lesion in question but also on the neurological status of the patient, whether it be cord, conus, or cauda injury, complete or incomplete.

STABLE INJURY/NEUROLOGICAL STATUS INTACT

Stable injuries with no neurologic deficit would encompass the anterior wedge, lateral wedge, or burst compression-type fracture. Surgery for the acute injury is not indicated. Analgesics for pain along with bed rest for a few days is usually sufficient. Occasionally the use of a body jacket is helpful. Follow-up from compression fractures of the spine demonstrates that 25% of these patients are asymptomatic, 55% have mild discomfort, and 20% have enough symptoms to produce some disability (22). Although the burst fracture was once believed to be stable, this is a relative distinction. We have noted that chronic instability may be evident and the spine may show a tendency to angulate, especially if the vertebral body comminution has been extensive. Therefore spine fusion may be indicated, but only as a late salvage procedure for persistent, incapacitating pain or progressive angulation and deformity.

STABLE INJURY/NEUROLOGIC DEFICIT

Stable injuries with neurologic deficit require a careful but realistic approach. Persistent interruption of spinal cord function over 24 hr is not benefited by surgery directed at reversing the neurological deficit. Treatment should be directed toward the patient's rehabilitation as a paraplegic. It is not justified to perform a laminectomy or any other "decompressive" procedure in order to assure the family that the patient "had everything done that was possible." Not only is this approach without documented benefit, but the unroofing procedure may produce spinal instability, converting a stable injury into an unstable one. If the patient has a stable injury and is paraplegic, there is no need for a stabilizing operation. On the other hand, if the injury is an incomplete cord lesion or lesion involving the cauda equina, significant functional neurologic improvement may result. We feel the improvement is often more substantial if any bony impingement on the neural tissues is removed. The impingement in these cases is almost invariably anterior, and therefore decompression must be directed at removing the anterior compression. Adequate reduction of the fracture may remove this bony impingement, but it is often difficult to accomplish since the fracture fragments may be comminuted and rigidly impacted. To remove this bone and perform an adequate anterior decompression, the approach may be anterior through a transthoracic, thoracoabdominal, or retroperitoneal incision. Once the comminuted bony fragments are removed from the spinal canal and neural elements, an anterior fusion, using rib or iliac bone as a strut graft, is essential. If the stability has been jeopardized by this approach and the anterior fusion does not provide sufficient stability, a posterior fusion with Harrington instrumentation should be carried out 2 weeks later. The anterior decompression may also be done through a posterolateral Capener-type approach, removing the facet joint and portion of the lamina with pedicle, providing access to the bony fragments that are pushing on the dura anteriorly. If this approach is used, however, the spine must be stabilized and a fusion carried out, since increased instability is produced by this approach, and further angulation may result.

UNSTABLE INJURIES WITH OR WITHOUT NEUROLOGIC DEFICIT

Unstable lesions with or without neurological deficit should be managed by open reduction of the fracture, internal fixation, and spine fusion. Untreated, these injuries may further displace, resulting in neurologic damage, increased instability, progressive deformity, and disabling back pain. Closed reduction alone of these fractures may lead to neurologic damage (22). For the operative approach to be most effective, it is best performed within 1 week of the injury or certainly before 3 to 4 weeks. Prior to surgery, the patient should be managed on a Foster or a horizontal Stryker turning frame. Vertical turning circle electric beds are contraindicated, since axial loading of the spine may result in severe displacement of the bony fragments. An unstable lesion with neurologic deficit requires attention to the fracture as well as to the neurologic status of the patient. We believe that anatomical realignment of the fracture remains the most certain method of decompressing the neural elements (Fig. 2). In unstable fractures associated with

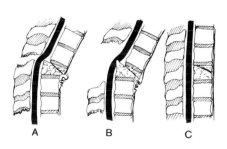

A   B   C

FIG. 2. Unstable injuries with or without neurological deficit must be stabilized to prevent late deformity and pain. Open reduction and internal fixation of the fracture is an effective method of accomplishing this objective. Laminectomy **(B)** does not decompress the neural elements completely but may lead to greater deformity. Anatomical realignment **(C)** of the spine not only furnishes optimal conditions for healing the fracture but also is an effective method of decompressing the neural elements.

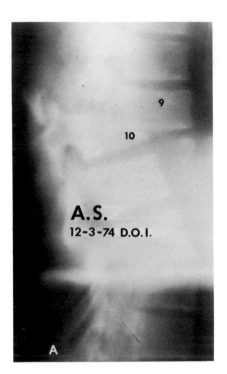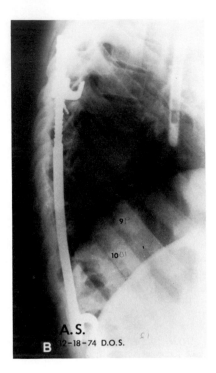

FIG. 3. A severely displaced unstable fracture as demonstrated, may be well reduced and the reduction maintained by the use of Harrington rods.

incomplete cord lesions or fractures involving the cauda, a limited laminectomy carried out in conjunction with fracture alignment and internal fixation can ensure removal of loose bony fragments and disc material and facilitate inspection for adequacy of reduction. If the neurologic deficit is complete, however, attention need only be given to aligning the fracture and ensuring stability by surgical arthrodesis (Fig. 3A,B). For unstable lesions with an incomplete neurologic deficit where treatment has been delayed for more than 3 to 4 weeks, complete reduction of the fracture may not be possible by the posterior approach. In these cases, there is still an anterior stepoff or bony impingement against the cord anteriorly. Here we favor an anterior cord decompression and an anterior spine fusion through a transthoracic, thoracoabdominal approach as necessary (Fig. 4A–D). A posterior spine fusion with instrumentation would be necessary if the stability achieved during the anterior fusion was not believed to be sufficient.

APPROACH

Following the injury, adequate x-rays and particularly tomography are most helpful. Myelography is sometimes thought to be beneficial, but as a routine procedure we have not found it particularly helpful, except in those cases where the neurologic deficit does not correlate anatomically with the level of bony injury. Once the presence of instability and/or neurologic deficit has been determined, the decision is made for surgical stabilization. The role of emergency surgery (within 24 hr) following acute spinal injury associated with a neurologic deficit is a controversial one at best. We believe that, except in those patients with a progressive neurologic deficit or a compound injury, decompression or stabilizing procedures should be delayed until the patient's condition is stabilized and adequate preoperative evaluation is completed. During this period of time, the patient should be managed on a horizontal turning frame, reducing the fracture as well as possible by positioning alone.

After the patient is stabilized, preferably within a few days after injury, he is taken to the operating room and carefully turned to a four-poster frame, allowing the spine to go into some extension without compression on the abdominal cavity. Through a midline incision over the area of the fracture/ dislocation, the spine is carefully exposed. The intraspinous ligament will be found disrupted with a large hematoma throughout the area. The exposure should proceed from two vertebra above the fracture/dislocation to two vertebrae below. The facet joint should be carefully cleaned out and a No. 1251 sharp cutting Harrington hook placed under the lamina on each side of the spinous processes two vertebrae above the fracture/dislocation. After the slot has been appropriately cut, a dull No. 1253 hook or a special ratcheted hook (No. 1262) may then be placed into the slot previously cut by the sharp-ended hook. A laminotomy is done over the lamina two vertebrae below to accept a No. 1254 hook underneath the lamina. The appropriate size Harrington rod is then placed between the two hooks on each side of the spinous processes and, by carefully levering the rod into the lower hooks, excellent fracture alignment and reduction of the fracture/dislocation is achieved. No attempt is made to distract the fracture fragments more than is consistent with restoring anatomy as it existed prior to the fracture/dislocation (Fig. 5A–C).

If there is any tendency to overdistraction, an 18-gauge wire may be placed around the spinous processes at the fracture/dislocation site and snugged together, preventing overdistraction from occurring. Although the rods are referred to as distracting rods, distraction is actually a misnomer, since anatomical realignment is all one is achieving and not distraction of the spine. We recommend decortication with a rongeurs and obtaining an iliac bone graft at the same time, placing bone chips over the area to be fused. If a posterolateral, Capener-type approach has been used to furnish anterior decompression, the area of the dura should be protected with gelfoam gauze and bone grafts placed lateral to the Harrington rods. The bony fusion area should be drained with a Hemovac catheter at the completion of the procedure and the wound closed in a customary fashion.

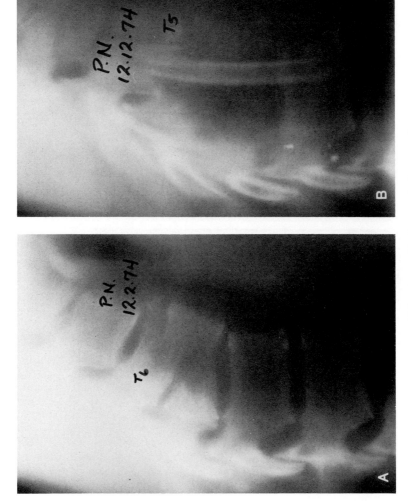

FIG. 4A–B. *(See legend facing page.)*

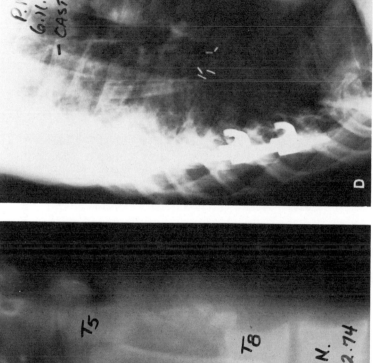

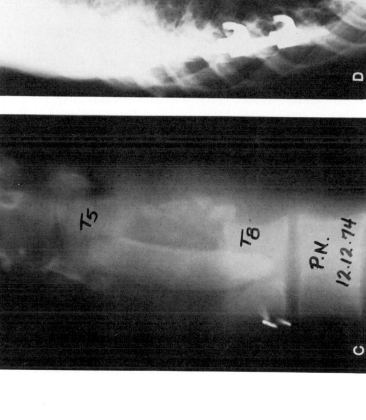

FIG. 4. A displaced flexion compression injury such as this with an incomplete neurological deficit has a favorable prognosis (**A**). A better neurological return may be anticipated if anterior decompression and fusion is carried out. Following anterior (transthoracic) decompression and fusion with an anterior rib strut graft (**B** and **C**), posterior instrumentation and fusion is carried out at a second stage 2 weeks later to ensure greater stability. The patient had only useless motor function in the lower extremities prior to surgery, and at the time of cast removal months later had regained complete neurological return (**D**).

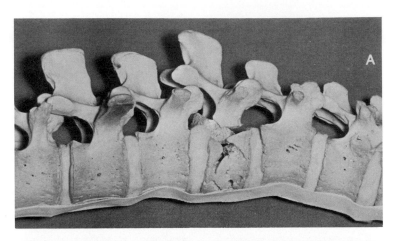

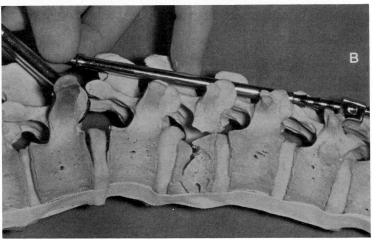

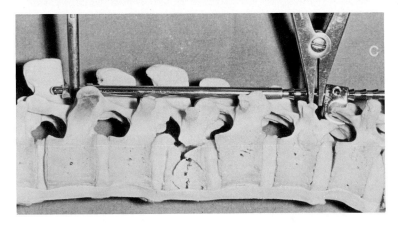

If the patient had a partial neurological deficit prior to surgery or even if the patient was neurologically intact, we recommend the "wake-up" test, i.e., having the anesthesiologist wake the patient after the rods have been placed *in situ* and instruct him to move his feet to command. This may be done safely while the patient is still intubated and provides immediate knowledge as to the neurological status of the patient after instrumentation is completed. It is a useful method of spinal cord monitoring; it is clinically applicable and, in our experience, is associated with no significant risk.

After completion of the procedure, the patient may be log-rolled in bed. The Hemovac catheter is removed at approximately 48 hr. Preoperative, intraoperative, and postoperative antibiotics are used routinely for 48 hr. Approximately 1 week after surgery, the patients are begun on rehabilitation. Those who are neurologically intact are placed in a body jacket; those with a neurological deficit are placed in a bivalved polypropylene body jacket, which may be easily removed every 2 to 4 hr for skin inspection. External immobilization is continued for approximately 4 to 6 months until the fusion appears solid.

One may ask, and logically so, whether (a) a more urgent approach should be taken to these injuries, especially in those with incomplete neurologic deficits; (b) is fusion really necessary; and (c) are all unstable fractures without significant displacement best managed in this fashion? Although some authors do feel that these fractures should be reduced immediately, the results in terms of neurologic return for incomplete lesions or in terms of fracture alignment do not appear significantly better than in those patients operated within 1 week. Spine fusion does not appear to be essential. However, once the fracture has healed, the Harrington rod or internal fixation device must eventually be removed, which requires a second operation. We believe that the fusion adds so little to the operative approach that the possibility of saving the patient a second operation justifies its performance.

It is certainly true that some patients with unstable fractures without displacement (especially those with fractures and minimal displacement in the thoracic spine that are splinted by the rib cage) might obtain satisfactory results from conservative management. Many of these injuries, however, do remain liable to further angulation. If the patient does have a complete neurologic deficit, a trial of conservative treatment with close radiological scrutiny is certainly reasonable. Any tendency for the spine to deform constitutes an indication for open reduction and internal fixation.

Although we favor the use of internal fixation instrumentation of the Har-

FIG. 5. Technique of open reduction and internal fixation using the Harrington distraction rod. The pathology is visualized **(A)**, and the appropriate hooks are placed in the facets two levels above and under the laminae two levels below, and the rod is secured in place **(B)**. Distraction is carried out only enough to reduce the fracture anatomically **(C)**. The fracture must not be overdistracted, and as a rule the intact anterior longitudinal ligament prevents this from developing. If a tendency for this to occur is apparent, the spinous processes may be wired together.

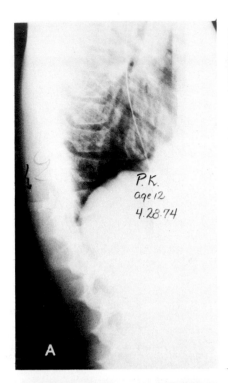

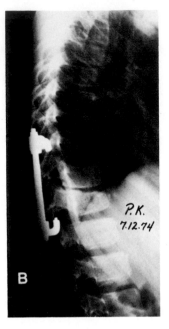

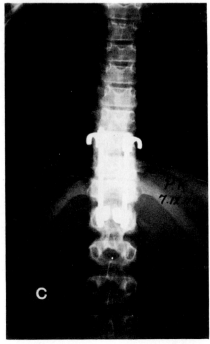

FIG. 6. The compression device may prove useful especially in the chance fracture (flexion, distraction) **(A)** with disruption of the interspinous ligament and locked facets. The compression device may facilitate excellent reduction with maintenance of stability **(B and C).**

rington distraction type, compression rods sometimes prove beneficial. We found compression devices particularly useful in patients with unstable kyphosis, particularly of the thoracic spine, where the posterior cortex of the vertebral body is not comminuted (Fig. 6A–C). However, if there is severe comminution, compression serves only to promote further extrusion of bony fragments posteriorly into the spinal canal. On the other hand, patients with Chance fractures or distraction-tension-type injuries that resulted in dislocation of the posterior facets may be conveniently managed by open reduction, facetectomy, and internal fixation with Harrington compression rods. Again, a spine fusion is recommended.

RESULTS

From our experience, which now consists of more than 80 patients managed by spine fusion and Harrington rod instrumentation for unstable fractures of the thoracic and lumbar spine, we have been impressed with the ease of reduction of these fractures, the decreased morbidity, the ease of rehabilitation, the decreased nursing care, and the early mobilization of the patients. Furthermore, the late complications from gibbus deformity and pain appear to be greatly lessened. Among our first 40 patients reviewed from 1964 to 1974 (9), 35 had a neurologic deficit and 5 were neurologically intact. No patient was made neurologically worse by the procedure, and 21 of the 23 patients with incomplete neurologic deficits improved after treatment. We made no attempt to attribute this exclusively to the reduction and internal fixation of the fracture, since (a) these patients were treated by a variety of surgical methods prior to spine stabilization, and (b) our experience is that incomplete lesions for the most part carry a favorable prognosis for some neurologic recovery. It has been gratifying, however, to note a definite decrease in the time of rehabilitation, which now averages 60 days for patients with complete lesions and 50 days for those with incomplete lesions treated by spine fusion and Harrington instrumentation.

SPECIAL PROBLEMS: PARAPLEGIA IN CHILDREN

Fractures of the spine in children, in contradistinction to those in the adult, have a different prognosis and require a different plan of management. Stable vertebral fractures in children unassociated with a neurological deficit rarely if ever result in progressive or delayed angulatory deformity. This is particularly true in those stable fractures that occur prior to age 10. Multiple compression fractures in children have a remarkable tendency to heal spontaneously and ultimately result in complete restoration of vertebral height. Indeed, rarely if ever are changes suggestive of Scheuermann's disease present over the vertebra initially injured. Lateral wedge fractures may result in minimal scoliosis but, again, progressive spine deformity is rarely

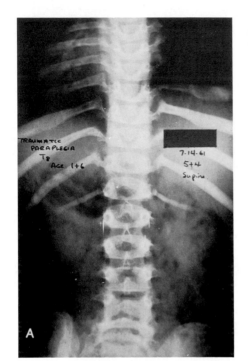
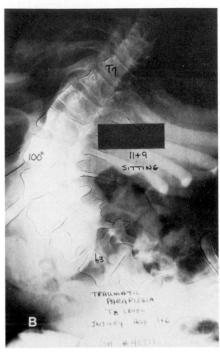
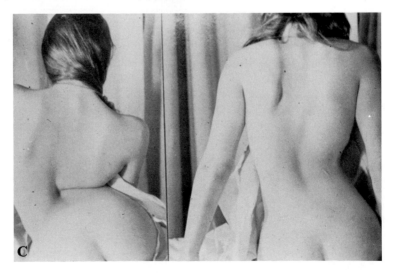

FIG. 7A–C. (*See legend facing page.*)

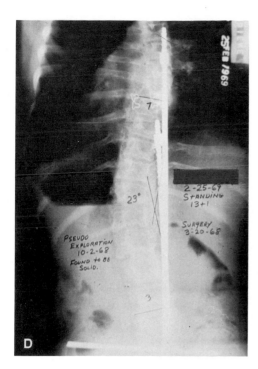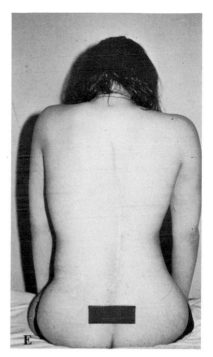

FIG. 7. This 5-year-old patient sustained a traumatic paraplegia at age 1 year l 0 months. Untreated, at age 11, a severe structural scoliosis is evident. Pre-operatively, the collapsing spine is evident, partially correctable by gravity (distraction) **(C)**. Extensive spine fusion with Harrington rod instrumentation was necessary **(D)**. Post-op result is satisfactory, freeing her upper extremities from trunk support **(E)**.

observed. This favorable prognosis is best explained by the absence of severe damage to the growth zone of the vertebral bodies at the time of the initial injury (2,19,20). This is in marked contrast to the unstable fracture dislocations that occur in children or those lesions of the spine associated with paraplegia or quadriplegia. The classical report by Kilfoyle et al. (23) and the experience developed at Rancho Los Amigos Hospital over the past 15 years demonstrates conclusively that patients who sustain a spinal cord injury prior to the adolescent growth spurt develop a spine deformity 100% of the time. This deformity may be lordosis, scoliosis, kyphosis, or a combination of all of these. We found this a predictable pattern also, one which unfortunately continues to occur too often (Fig. 7A–E). Therefore children sustaining a traumatic paraplegia prior to the adolescent growth spurt (i.e., approximately age 10 in the female and age 12 in the male) should be braced until the completion of growth. The bivalve polypropylene body jacket is an excellent orthosis and serves to stabilize an unstable collapsing spine, allowing easy removal and easy application. Spine fusion with in-

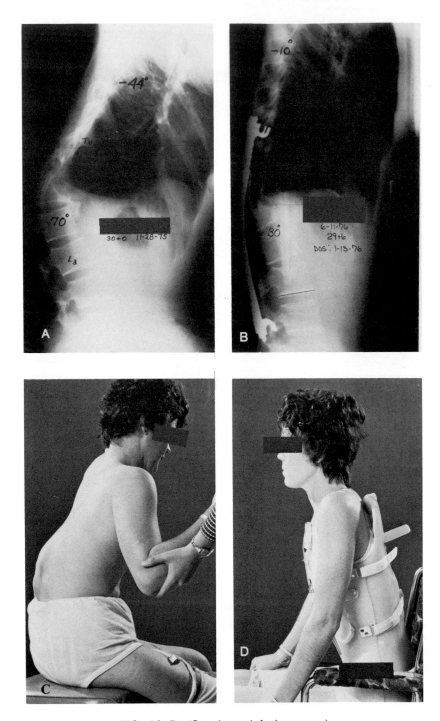

FIG. 8A–D. (*See legend facing page.*)

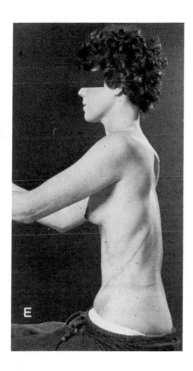

FIG. 8. This patient sustained a complete T11 paraplegia, undergoing a laminectomy within 24 to 48 hr post injury. The kyphosis has steadily progressed for two years resulting in pain, pressure ulceration, and instability to maintain sitting balance **(A)**. An anterior fusion using a fibula graft followed two weeks later by posterior Harrington rods has resulted in a maintained and stable correction **(B)**. Pre-op **(C)**, immediate post-op in brace **(D)**, 8 months post-op **(E)**.

strumentation is indicated for those patients with progressive deformity uncontrolled by bracing during the growth period or those patients presenting with significant deformity after growth is complete. Spine fusion with Harrington instrumentation is the procedure of choice, and the fusion should extend all the way to the sacrum. Failure to include the sacrum results in progressive pelvic obliquity, loss of sitting balance, and pressure ulceration over the buttocks from unequal weight distribution applied to the ischium.

LATE KYPHOSIS SECONDARY TO TRAUMATIC SPINE DEFORMITY

Those patients presenting with chronic instability or progressive angular deformity of the spine, either from untreated fracture/dislocation initially or from fractures treated by laminectomy resulting in greater instability, require surgical arthrodesis. The problem is primarily one of traumatic kyphosis, and if the kyphosis is greater than 50° to 60°, an anterior interbody or strut graft fusion is necessary to supplement the posterior arthrodesis. The decision of whether to do the anterior fusion first or the posterior fusion first depends on the structural nature of the kyphosis. If the kyphosis is supple and nonstructural, easily correctable on hyperextension, then a posterior fusion might be done first with an anterior interbody fusion following 2 weeks later. If the kyphosis is rigid, however, an anterior fusion should be carried out as the first step in order to loosen up and allow correction of the fixed deformity. The procedure is completed with insertion of a rib or fibular strut graft, followed 2 weeks later by posterior arthrodesis with Harrington rod instrumentation (Fig. 8A–E). Those patients presenting during adulthood with progressive scoliosis associated with severe structural pelvic obliquity may be managed successfully also with the Dwyer instrumentation through the anterior approach. However, posterior arthrodesis with Harrington instrumentation must always be carried out with extension of the fusion to the sacrum. Otherwise, pelvic obliquity occurs and correction is lost.

SUMMARY

Injuries to the thoracic and lumbar spine may result in severe instability with progressive neurologic deficit. Attention must be directed not only to restoring or improving neurologic function where possible, but also to promoting bony stability, preventing catastrophic late complications of angular deformity, pressure ulceration, skin breakdown, and progressive neurologic deficit. Early stabilization of unstable lesions by spine fusion and Harrington instrumentation has been shown to be beneficial in restoring spinal alignment, allowing early mobilization of the patient, shortening rehabilitation, and preventing the late complications of increasing deformity with incapacitating pain.

REFERENCES

1. Albee, F. (1940): *Bone Graft Surgery*. Appleton, New York.
2. Aufdermaur, M. (1974): Spinal injuries in juveniles: Necropsy findings twelve cases. *J. Bone Joint Surg.*, 56B:513.
3. Bedbrook, G. M. (1969): Use and disuse of surgery in lumbo-dorsal fractures. *J. Western Pacific Orthop. Assoc.*, VI:S–26.
4. Bradford, D. S., Akbarnia, B., Winter, R. B., and Seljeskog, E. (1977): *Surgical Treatment of Fracture and Fracture Dislocations of the Thoracic Spine (in press)*.
5. Bradford, D. S., and Thompson, R. C. (1976): Fractures and dislocations of the spine: Indications for surgical intervention. *Minn. Med.*, 59:711.
6. Brown, C. W., Odom, J. A., Donaldson, D. H., and Cvong, T. V. (1976): Weiss spring instrumentation for fracture dislocation of the spine with associated neurologic deficit. *Proceedings, Scoliosis Research Society, 11th Annual Meeting*, Ottawa.
7. Dick, I. L. (1953): The treatment of traumatic paraplegia in fractures of the lumbo-dorsal spine. *Edinburgh Med. J.*, 60:249.
8. Dickinson, J. H., Harrington, P. R., and Erwin, W. D. (1973): Harrington instrumentation in the fractured, unstable thoracic and lumbar spine. *Texas Med.*, 69:91–98.
9. Flesch, J. R., Leider, L. L., Erickson, D. L., Chou, S. N., and Bradford, D. S. (1977): Harrington instrumentation and spine fusion for thoracic and lumbar spine fractures. *J. Bone Joint Surg. (in press)*.
10. Frankel, H. L., Hancock, D. O., Hyslop, G., Melzak, J., Michaelis, L. S., Ungar, G. H., Vernon, J. D. S., and Walsh, J. J. (1969): The value of postural reduction in the initial management of closed injuries of the spine with paraplegia and tetraplegia. *Paraplegia*, 7:179.

11. Guttmann, L. (1949): Surgical aspects of the treatment of traumatic paraplegia. *J. Bone Joint Surg.*, 31B:339.
12. Guttmann, L. (1954): Initial treatment of traumatic paraplegia. *Proc. R. Soc. Med.*, 47: 1103–1109.
13. Guttmann, I.. (1969): Spinal deformities in traumatic paraplegia and tetraplegics following surgical procedures. *Paraplegia*, 7:38–58.
14. Hardy, A. G. (1965): The treatment of paraplegia due to dislocations of the dorso-lumbar spine. *Paraplegia*, 3:112–119.
15. Harrington, P. R. (1967): Instrumentation in spine instability other than scoliosis. *South Afr. J. Surg.*, 5:7–12.
16. Harrington, P. R. (1972): Technical details in relation to the successful use of instrumentation in scoliosis. *Orthop. Clin. North Am.*, 3:49–67.
17. Holdsworth, F. W., and Hardy, A. (1953): Early treatment of paraplegia from fractures of the thoracolumbar spine. *J. Bone Joint Surg.*, 35B:540–550.
18. Hone, M., and Cornish, B. (1969): Personal communication, 1968. Cited by Bedbrook, G. M.: Use and disuse of surgery in lumbo-dorsal fractures. *J. Western Pacific Orthop. Assoc.*, VI:5–26.
19. Horal, J., Nachemson, A., and Scheller, S. (1972): Clinical and radiological long term follow-up of vertebral fractures in children. *Acta Orthop. Scand.*, 43:491.
20. Hubbard, D. D. (1974): Injuries of the spine in children and adolescents, *Injuries Spine*, 100:56.
21. Katznelson, A. M. (1969): Stabilization of the spine in traumatic paraplegia. *Paraplegia*, 7:33–37.
22. Kaufer, H. (1972): The thoracolumbar spine. In: *Fractures*, edited by Charles A. Rockwood, Jr. and David P. Green. Lippincott, Philadelphia.
23. Kilfoyle, R. M., Foley, J. J., and Norton, P. L. (1965): Spine and pelvic deformity in childhood and adolescent paraplegia. *J. Bone Joint Surg.*, 47A:659.
24. Lewis, J., and McKibben, B. (1974): The treatment of unstable fracture-dislocations of the thoraco-lumbar spine accompanied by paraplegia. *J. Bone Joint Surg.*, 56B:603.
25. Mullen, M. P., Grenn, D. R., and Tupper, J. W. (1976): Early experience with Weiss spinal spring instrumentation for unstable fractures and other spinal deformities. *Proceedings, Scoliosis Research Society 11th Annual Meeting*, Ottawa.
26. Nicoll, E. A. (1949): Fractures of the dorso-lumbar spine. *J. Bone Joint Surg.*, 31B:376.
27. Pennybacker, J. B. (1953): The treatment of traumatic paraplegia. *J. Bone Joint Surg.*, 35B:517.
28. Roberts, J. B., and Curtiss, P. H. (1970): Stability of the thoracic and lumbar spine in traumatic paraplegia following fracture of fracture dislocation. *J. Bone Joint Surg.*, 52A: 115–1130.
29. Woodburne, R. T. (1957): *Essentials of Human Anatomy*. Oxford University Press, New York.

Spinal Deformities and Neurological Dysfunction, edited by S. N. Chou and E. L. Seljeskog. Raven Press, New York © 1978.

Spondylolysis and Spondylolisthesis

David S. Bradford

Department of Orthopedic Surgery, University of Minnesota, Minneapolis, Minnesota 55455

Spondylolisthesis is defined as a slipping forward of one vertebra on another. The origin of this word comes from Greek *spondylos,* meaning vertebra, and *olisthesis,* meaning to slip. Recognition of this condition began with the work of Herbiniaux (16), a Belgian obstetrician who noted in 1782 that there were times when a bony prominence in front of the sacrum caused problems in delivery. He is generally credited with having first described the complete dislocation of the body of L5 over in front of the sacrum. The term spondylolisthesis was coined by Killian in 1854 (18) who believed that the lesion was caused by slow subluxation of the lumbosacral facets. One year later Robert (36) noted the location of the lesion to be in the pars interarticularis. Neugebauer in 1881 (29) was the first to recognize that a slippage between L5 and sacrum can occur by elongation of the pars interarticularis, without a break in continuity. Lambl in 1858 (20) was the first to be credited with demonstrating the actual discontinuity of that portion of the neural arch known as the pars interarticularis, a defect in the neural arch, now referred to as spondylolysis.

DESCRIPTION AND ETIOLOGY

The following classification represents the most recent one published and has been derived from previous classifications reported by Wiltse et al. (48) (Fig. 1):

Dysplastic: In this type of spondylolisthesis, congenital abnormalities in the upper sacrum in the arch of L5 permit forward slippage to L5.

Isthmic: This is a lesion of the pars interarticularis in which three types can be identified: (a) lytic or fatigue fracture of the pars; (b) elongated but intact pars; (c) acute fracture.

Degenerative: Secondary to longstanding degenerative arthritis and intersegmental instability of the facet joints.

Traumatic: Secondary to fractures in areas of the bony hook other than the pars.

Pathological: Here there is generalized or localized bone disease (Paget's, etc.).

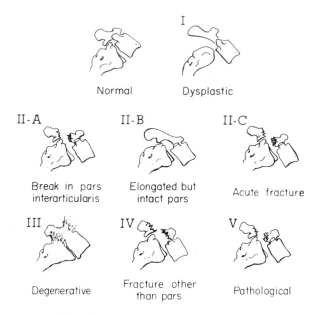

FIG. 1. Classification of spondylolisthesis.

Dysplastic Spondylolisthesis

In the dysplastic type of spondylolisthesis, there is a congenital dysplasia of the upper sacrum and/or the neural arch of L5. This creates insufficient bony stock to withstand the forward thrust of the lumbar spine, and therefore the L5 lumbar vertebra gradually slips forward on the sacrum. The pars interarticularis may remain unchanged, but if it does the slippage cannot exceed more than 25% with cauda equina paralysis. Usually, however, the pars either elongates or fractures, making it difficult to tell this type from type IIA or IIB (Fig. 2). In surgery, however, the abnormal relationships are readily apparent. There is almost invariably a spina bifida of the sacrum, and the L5 vertebra may also show a wide spina bifida. This type usually goes on to a severe grade of slippage and appears, according to Wiltse et al., to be twice as common in females as males (48).

Isthmic Spondylolisthesis

In the isthmic type of spondylolisthesis, the basic defect is in the pars interarticularis. *Subtype A* is a fracture of the pars and is almost always secondary to a stress or fatigue fracture (Fig. 2). This is the most common type in persons under age 50 and is rarely seen in those under age 5. It is never seen at birth, and the youngest patient, reported by Borkow and Kleiger (4), was 4 months of age. The incidence of the defect in adult

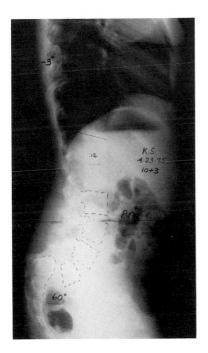
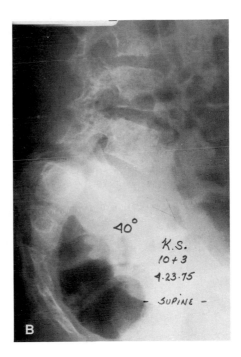

FIG. 2. Severity of the spondylolisthesis may be greater than appreciated when the supine x-ray is compared with the standing. In **2B**, a dysplastic type, which has developed elongation of the pars with ultimate lysis is apparent.

Caucasian Americans appears to be approximately 5 to 6% (3). Steward (42) found that Eskimos have by far the highest incidence, as high as 50% in isolated communities north of the Yukon. It should also be noted that there is approximately 30% incidence of spondylolisthesis in members of families of affected individuals (3,46). It is also of interest that spina bifida is 13 times more frequent in patients with spondylolisthesis than in the general population. It is the opinion of many authors (10,26,31,49) that isthmic spondylosis is a result of fatigue fractures from repeated trauma and stress, rather than from any one acute traumatic episode. However, it differs from other fatigue fractures in the following respects. It tends to develop at an earlier age; there is a hereditary predisposition; callus formation is rarely seen and the defect in the pars tends to persist, although occasional healing may occur. In this regard, it is of interest that female gymnasts have a four times higher incidence of spondylolysis than their nonathletic female peers (18). It is not known whether these stress fractures are due to flexion or extension stresses. It is known, however, that it never occurs in animals of a lower order than man, and only man has a true lumbar lordosis and a true upright posture.

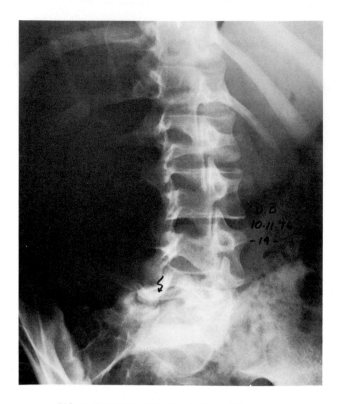

FIG. 3. Type IIB with elongation of the pars.

Subtype B is an elongation of the pars without separation (Fig. 3). This is fundamentally the same lesion as subtype A. It occurs secondary to repeated stress fractures which heal with the pars assuming a more elongated position as the body of L5 slides forward. Eventually it may separate as slippage continues to occur, making it difficult to differentiate from subtype A. The fundamental disease as well as the presumed etiology is the same.

Subtype C is an acute pars fracture. This is always secondary to severe trauma—usually, we believe, an extension-type fracture. Slippage rarely occurs; heredity does not seem to play a role in the etiology of this type.

Degenerative Spondylolisthesis

The degenerative type is probably the most common form of spondylolisthesis (Fig. 4). None of the affected patients are younger than age 40, and very few are younger than age 50. This type is four to five times more frequent in the female than in the male. Newman and Stone first gave this the descriptive title in 1963 (31), although previous authors had referred to it and recognized its significance some 30 years before. There is no pars

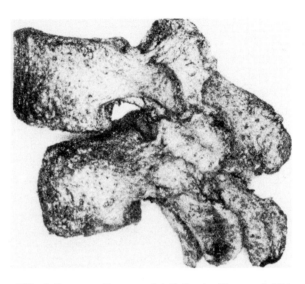

FIG. 4. Degenerative spondylolisthesis. (From ref. 38.)

interarticularis defect in this type, and the slippage is never greater than 30% unless the patient has undergone a laminectomy. Advanced degenerative disease of the facet joints and disc is the exclusive finding that separates this condition from the other types of spondylolisthesis. The L4–L5 area is affected more commonly than other levels, and sacralization of L5 is four times more frequent (38). The predisposing factor is thought to be a straight, stable lumbosacral joint, which puts increased stress on the intervertebral joint between L4 and L5, ultimately leading to hypermobility and degeneration of the articular processes and disc. Degenerative changes and the forward slipping combine to produce localized spinal stenosis which may compress the nerve roots of the cauda equina (38) (Fig. 5).

Traumatic Spondylolisthesis

The traumatic type of spondylolisthesis is secondary to an acute injury which fractures some part of the bony hook other than the pars interarticularis and allows forward slippage of the vertebrae. This is always due to severe trauma and usually heals with immobilization.

Pathological Spondylolisthesis

Generalized bone disease (e.g., Albers-Schonberg and arthrogryposis) may lead to fractures or elongation of the pars interarticularis. Paget's disease also has been associated with elongation of the pars and spondylolisthesis. Local factors such as fractures of the pars at the upper end of the

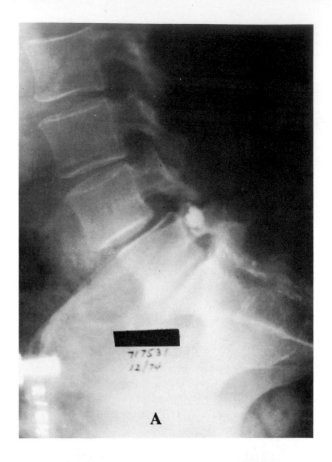

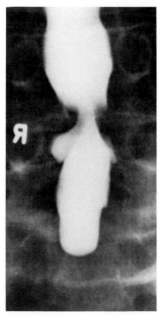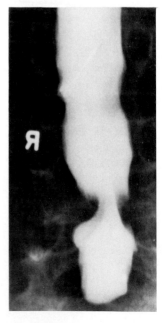

FIG. 5. Degenerative spondylolisthesis with forward slipping of L4 on L5 and an hour glass constriction noted on the myelogram.

lumbar fusion likewise have been reported. These are not common but are probably secondary to fatigue fracture from altered mechanics of the spine.

SIGNS AND SYMPTOMS: CHILDREN AND ADOLESCENTS

Spondylolisthesis in children behaves differently from that in adults. At least two types exist in children, producing pain in the back or legs or a combination of both. The types present as: (a) a defect in the pars with mild to moderate slip and backache predominating, with or without leg pain; (b) a high grade of slip (grade IV or V) with a typical spondylolisthesis build—a short torso and heart-shaped buttocks. Pain in the back (1) is probably secondary to instability of the affected segment that produced strain on the intervertebral ligaments and joints. This may ultimately lead to localized osteoarthritis. The pain may arise from disc degeneration, although herniation of the intervertebral disc is extremely uncommon. Pain also may arise from a defect in the pars, especially if there has been a fairly acute fracture. It should be emphasized that not every patient with spondylolysis or spondylolisthesis suffers from low back pain. We have seen patients with rather severe degrees of spondylolisthesis (75 to 100%) who are totally asymptomatic. In fact, it is felt by some authors (Nachemson, *personal communication*) that spondylolysis without spondylolisthesis is not associated with back pain in any greater incidence than among the general population. The second type of pain is due to pressure on the roots of the sacral plexus and is less common than backache. From the distorted anatomy created and the narrowing of the intervertebral foramen between the 5th lumbar and the first sacral vertebra, as well as the fibrocartilagenous callus of the fractured pars, pressure on the L5 root is produced. If the compression of the roots is severe, bilateral sciatica is evident. Compression can happen to other components of the cauda equina, i.e., the sacral roots which pass over the top of the sacrum that are compressed at this site by the forward displacement of the lumbar vertebrae above. This latter type of compression is far less common than the foraminal compression of the 5th root.

The deformity of spondylolisthesis is very characteristic (Fig. 6). It is secondary to the forward slippage of the involved vertebra. When it becomes quite severe (75 to 100%), compensating mechanisms are brought into play, and these must be recognized. As the vertebra slips forward, it leaves behind the lamina, spinous processes, and the inferior articular facets. Consequently, there is a step-off palpable over the spinous processes from the one left behind to the ones slipped above. As the vertebrae above are carried further forward, they displace the center of body gravity; to compensate for this, the lumbar spine above the lesion becomes hyperextended, and the upper part of the trunk is thrown further backward. In an attempt to realign the weight of the body and to support it more adequately, the pelvis becomes rotated about its transverse axis so that the sacrum actually be-

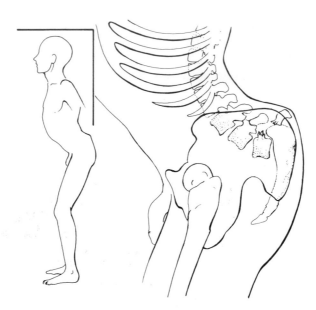

FIG. 6. Demonstrating the characteristic deformity of spondylolisthesis. Note that with severe deformity, the sacrum becomes almost vertical and the anterior superior iliac spine rides higher than the posterior superior iliac spine. Hip appears flexed even though it is fully extended in relation to the sacrum while the knee becomes truly flexed if the patient attempts to stand straight.

comes vertical (15). One can clearly see this by noting that the anterior superior spine rises to the same level or even becomes higher than the posterior superior spine (Fig. 6). The buttocks appear "heart-shaped" secondary to the sacral prominence. The hip joint rotates with the tilted pelvis until the thigh, even in extreme degrees of full extension, fails to place itself vertically underneath the trunk. Consequently, when the affected patient tries to stand straight, his hips remain flexed beneath his torso and the knees must also remain flexed in order to place the feet beneath the body. If he attempts to stand with his legs straight, the trunk must tilt forward at the hip since the hips cannot hyperextend enough to compensate for this. As the slip becomes greater, the trunk is severely shortened, so there is an almost complete absence of the waistline and the rib cage abuts the iliac crest. It is useful also to think of this as a flexion deformity or a "kyphosis" of L5 on S1, for not only is L5 forward-translated on S1 but forward-tilted as well. This disturbed anatomy, along with the associated hamstring tightness described by Phalen and Dickson (35), produces a peculiar yet characteristic gait.

These children often develop a functional scoliosis. This is also referred to as a "sciatic scoliosis" and is usually secondary to muscle spasm produced by irritation of the nerve roots. If the scoliosis is a sciatic-type scoliosis, it usually extends down to the sacrum. Idiopathic scoliosis may also be seen in association with spondylolisthesis, but it is usually thoracic or thoraco-lumbar and is not secondary to muscle spasm or nerve root irritation.

Neurologic evaluation may reveal nerve root impairment, particularly involving the L5 nerve roots. With severe degrees of neurologic involvement, bowel or bladder signs or symptoms may develop, although this is uncommon.

The progression of spondylolisthesis may be slow or quite rapid. Progressive degrees of slip often occur during periods of rapid growth or just at the late juvenile or early adolescent period.

SIGNS AND SYMPTOMS: ADULTS

The adult with degenerative spondylolisthesis experiences either back pain or a combination of back and leg pain. The back pain is rarely severe and often exists for several years with long periods of remission. Patients rarely associate their symptoms with activity, weather, or other discernible factors (38). Spinal stenosis-type symptoms (spinal claudication) are uncommon but when they occur are usually constant. These symptoms are often relieved by sitting or lying, in contrast to vascular claudication, which is usually relieved by standing in place. Radicular pain may be present. It is usually sensory in nature, but sometimes motor findings are evident.

DIAGNOSIS

With a well-marked deformity on physical examination, the diagnosis is rather simple. When the deformity is inconspicuous, adequate radiographic evaluation is essential. If there is a significant degree of slippage, a lateral x-ray reveals the defect and the percentage of slip. Meyerding (25) classified the percentage of slippage accordingly: grade I 0 to 25%; grade II 25 to 50%; grade III 50 to 75%; grade IV >75%. If the gap at the defect is slight and there is no forward displacement, oblique radiographic projections are essential. Laminography is also helpful. In the anterior/posterior projection, a severe deformity may be visualized from the outline and appearance of the body of L5 as it slips forward, making a characteristic picture referred to as Napoleon's hat. In cases of degenerative spondylolisthesis, the radiographic findings are characteristic: Degenerative joint disease can be visualized, and a slippage of L4 on L5 is evident without a defect in the pars interarticularis. Disc space narrowing is usual. It should also be noted that standing x-rays in the lateral position are extremely valuable. Although supine x-rays may show a slippage, standing x-rays often show the slippage to be much greater than would be appreciated on the supine film (Fig. 2). This was noted by Lowe et al. (24), and it has been our experience as well.

We therefore recommend recumbent and standing lateral lumbosacral spine x-rays to compare the mobility of the slip as well as its true magnitude. Hyperextension and hyperflexion x-rays are also useful for determining mobility. Preoperative evaluation may also include a myelogram to evaluate the status of the exiting lumbar nerve root at the site of the anticipated impingement. Extrusion of an intervertebral disc may occur at or adjacent to the level of the spondylolisthesis, thus impairing function of corresponding nerve roots. It is our experience that disc herniation in association with spondylolisthesis is extremely uncommon; from reports in the literature, it appears to be less than 5% (22). We do not perform myelography as a routine procedure. In severe degrees of slippage (>75%), a complete block of the myelogram is characteristic but does not imply compression of neural tissues. In the adult with degenerative spondylolisthesis unresponsive to conservative management, however, we recommend myelography as a routine procedure prior to undertaking surgical intervention.

TREATMENT OF SPONDYLOLYSIS

Children

Although spondylolysis usually originates at age 5 to 10 years with an incidence approaching 5%, few of these patients are symptomatic. Those who respond, for the most part, respond to simple conservative measures. We do not believe that asymptomatic patients or those with minimal symptoms need to limit their activity. Repeated x-ray evaluation at 6-month intervals is advisable in those patients less than 10 years of age. A small percentage of patients with persistent symptoms that do not repond to conservative measures may require surgical stabilization with a lateral process fusion from L5 to sacrum. Extension of the fusion to L4 is not necessary. There is no indication for a Gill procedure or a wide laminectomy. It should be stressed that symptomatic spondylolysis in the adolescent is most uncommon, and one should rule out other causes of back pain in children (i.e., infection, tumor, osteoid osteoma, herniated disc) before surgery is undertaken.

Adults

Conservative treatment for the adult with a lytic spondylolisthesis is the same as that for backache due to other causes. Heat, analgesics, exercises, anti-inflammatory medication, along with a corset or body jacket may be tried with some degree of success. For persistent pain unresponsive to conservative management, spine fusion should be performed. Myelography should be done and disc herniation surgically removed if indicated. Generally for patients under 50 years of age, we prefer spinal arthrodesis as the treatment of choice. Patients over 50 can usually be managed by laminectomy alone. Surgery is carried out primarily for the relief of pain and not to prevent progression of the slip. The slip rarely increases to a significant degree in the adult, and if slippage does develop it may be managed by posterolateral spine fusion.

TREATMENT OF SPONDYLOLISTHESIS

Dysplastic and Isthmic Type

Treatment of the child with spondylolisthesis depends to a large part on the severity of symptoms and the degree of slippage. If the symptoms are minimal and the slip is less than 25%, conservative treatment consisting of routine back care, general abdominal strengthening exercises, and a temporary lumbar sacral corset may prove helpful. Persistent symptoms unresponsive to conservative management and interfering with normal childhood activities necessitate surgical management. The need for operative intervention rests not only on the severity of symptoms but also on the degree of slippage. Further slipping may occur in the child but almost never in the adult; and if the L5 vertebral body is trapezoid in shape and the upper end of the sacrum has assumed a dome-shaped, somewhat vertical orientation, there is greater than a 50% likelihood that the patient will have progressive slippage (44,45) If the slippage continues to progress past 25% or if the child is symptomatic, spine fusion is indicated. It is our belief that the fusion should be performed in the growing child before the displacement exceeds one-third the length of the vertebral body. Certainly, if the displacement is more than 50%, even if the child has no symptoms, spine fusion is indicated (23,28,32,47). Any child in whom a defect is discovered early, especially under age 10, should have lateral standing roentgenograms of the lumbosacral area taken every 6 months until the completion of growth. This is particularly important in females because a high grade of slippage is twice as common in girls as in boys (47). Surgery in the child consists of spine fusion with or without decompression by laminectomy (Fig. 7). Laminectomy (12) (Gill procedure) as an isolated procedure in a growing child is contraindicated (28). Further slippage with laminectomy alone occurs in a high percentage of cases (22,28). The most effective treatment is lumbosacral fusion, and we recommend extending the fusion from L4 to the sacrum. The fusion should be done posterolaterally; it may be done through a midline incision, through a paraspinal approach, splitting the sacrospinalis muscle approximately two fingerbreadths lateral to the midline, or an approach lateral to the paraspinal muscles. Fusion should extend out to the tips of the transverse processes from L4 down to the sacral alae, using autogenous iliac bone for grafting. It may be quite difficult to reach

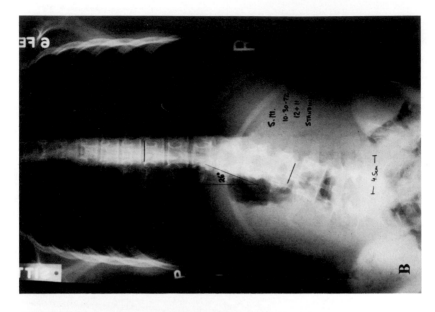

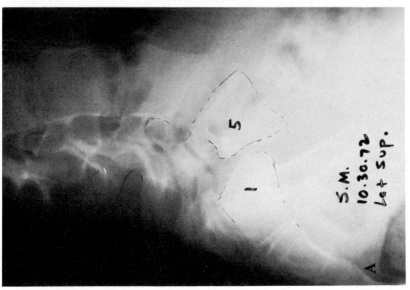

FIG. 7A–B. (See legend facing page.)

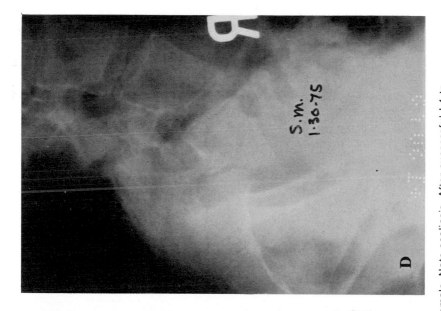

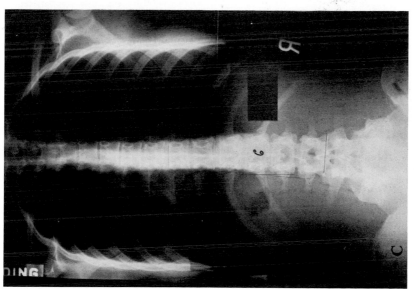

FIG. 7. Spondylolisthesis in a 12-year-old female. Note scoliosis. After successful L4 to sacrum fusion **(C,D)** scoliosis has disappeared.

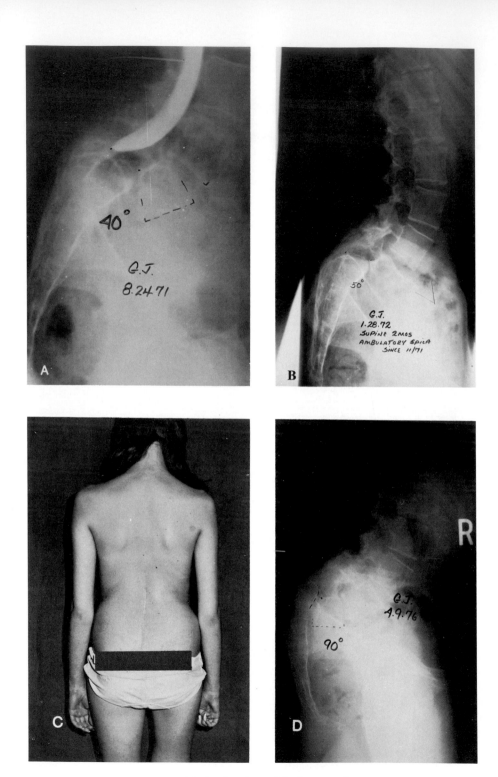

FIG. 8A–D. (*See legend facing page.*)

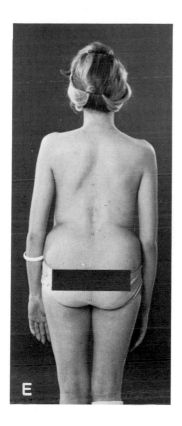

FIG. 8. This patient with a severe slip underwent a Gill and L4 to sacrum fusion on 9-1-71. She was kept down for 2 months in a pantaloon spica and ambulated for 2 weeks in a walking spica. Fusion looked solid on 1-28-72 **(B)** and clinical appearance satisfactory **(C)**. However, she continued to slip and last follow-up on 4-9-76 **(D and E)** shows an unsatisfactory cosmetic result. The fusion however, is solid.

the L5 transverse process in extreme degrees of slippage; therefore solidification of the fusion is more assured by extending the fusion to the transverse process of L4. The articular facet joints of L4 to L5 and L5 to S1 should be cleaned of articular cartilage and cancellous bone packed into the facet joint. There is some doubt about whether decompression with removal of loose posterior element of L5 should be done in children, irrespective of the signs and symptoms of neurologic compromise. In fact, it is the contention of Wiltse and Jackson (47) that severely tight hamstrings, decreased Achilles reflexes, and even a footdrop recover after a solid arthrodesis is effected. It is our belief, however, that if the patient has bowel or bladder symptoms, severe hamstring tightness, and/or a footdrop, a midline posterior approach with removal of the loose posterior element and fibrocartilagenous callus overlying the compressed L5 root should be done. Removal of the posterior superior prominence of the sacrum has also been suggested, but we have not found this necessary. It should be stressed that with all of these decompressive procedures spine stabilization by fusion, especially in children, must be undertaken.

Postoperatively, adult patients are encouraged to begin ambulation 1 to 2 days after surgery. Routine abdominal isometric and gluteal sitting exercises are started 2 to 4 days after the operation. Sitting in straight-backed rather than soft chairs is encouraged for the first 2 months after surgery, and patients are instructed to avoid excessive motion to the low back by rolling like a log instead of twisting, and by bending at the knees when stooping to pick up objects from the floor. Corsets and braces may be used but do not appear to be essential for a solid arthrodesis. In the adult, if slippage is greater than 50%, we prefer to keep the patient prone for approximately 5 to 7 days and then apply a body spica cast with a single thigh extension in order to facilitate greater immobilization of the lumbosacral spine and a more certain arthrodesis. The cast remains in place for 3 to 4 months following discharge from the hospital. The patient may be ambulatory.

In the child with a slip of 50% or more, we believe it best to use a body cast extending to both thighs with the hips in extension. The patient is kept in bed for 4 months, lessening the likelihood of further slippage.

Further slippage may occur after spine fusion, even if the patient is kept supine (Fig. 8). This has been noted by Newman (30), Bosworth et al. (5), Dandy and Shannon (7), and Laurent and Osterman (23). It is Wiltse and Jackson's contention that the use of the midline posterior approach may increase the instability and, even with a successful arthrodesis, permit further slippage. However, if a posterolateral approach is used, without removing the loose laminae, further slippage is less likely (47).

Alternatives in Management

Reduction of Spondylolisthesis

During the past 25 years, increasing attention has been given to the possibility of reducing the spondylolisthesis and then performing surgical arthrodesis, either posteriorly, anteriorly, or both. In 1951 Harris, proposed the principle that skeletal traction could indeed reduce spondylolisthesis (15). Newman in 1965 (30) described a method of reducing spondylolisthesis but believed that the reduction was never maintained during the period of consolidation of the posterior arthrodesis. Lance (21) reported successful reduction of the spondylolisthesis in 1966, and Harrington et al. later proposed the technique of open reduction and internal fixation with distracting devices for severe degrees of slippage (13,14). Other authors since then have developed alternative procedures for reducing the spondylolisthesis that look quite promising (9,39–41).

Particularly appealing is Scaglietti's technique for reduction of spondylolisthesis with casting. In this technique, the patient is placed on a fracture table and, following longitudinal distraction, the hips are hyperextended, actually reducing the spondylolisthesis and correcting the abnormal forward

TABLE 1. *Results of spine fusion; Harrington rod instrumentation for management of severe spondylolisthesis*

| Patient | Age/sex | % Slippage | | | Thoracic kyphosis (initial/1 yr) | Type of defect |
		Initial	During surgery	1 yr		
D.S.	11+2/F	60	21	37	0°/−17°	IIB
C.C.	12+3/F	40	0	10	30°/10°	I/IIB
R.B.	15+1/M	56	25	30	— —	I/IIB
K.S.	10+3/F	>100	78	78	−3°/−30	I/IIA
C.K.	11+10/F	>100	84	84	10°/−12	I/IIA/B

pelvic inclination. A plaster cast is then applied. The patient is kept in the plaster some 4 months before undergoing surgery, allowing reconstitution of the distorted anatomy. The second stage consists of a posterior spine fusion with internal instrumentation.

The Harrington technique consists of a spinal instrumentation from L1 to sacrum, using a modified sacral bar with posterior interbody fusion and a lateral gutter fusion from L3 to sacrum. We modified Harrington's technique and have used it on five patients since 1972 (Table 1). The technique consists of a posterior approach, instrumentation from T12 or L1 to sacrum, placing the lower hook on the sacral alar, bending the rod to maintain lumbar lordosis, removing the free floating posterior element of L5, decompression of the L5 root, and then performing a lateral process fusion from L4 to sacrum using an iliac bone graft. The patients are ambulated 1 week after surgery in a body cast; and the rod is removed 6 months postoperatively, after the fusion is solid (Fig. 9). Complications consisted of (a) facet subluxation at T12–L1, subsequently requiring open reduction and fusion of the facet between T12 and L1; and (b) a dislodged rod. No loss of correction occurred, however. Of concern is the loss of thoracic kyphosis and even the increase in pre-existing thoracic lordosis with this technique. Of great interest are the findings revealed at operation. After the posterior element is removed, the dura still remains tight and constricted without pulsations. Once distraction is carried out, pulsations appear and the L5 root becomes visualized as it becomes decompressed from the pars adjoining the superior facet of L5 and the pedicle (Fig. 10). In fact, the visual decompression achieved by this distraction and reduction technique is far greater than that achieved by the Gill procedure.

The question must be asked, however, whether this technique is safe and worth the effort. Complications may be minimal if the technique is performed properly. The clinical and cosmetic results achieved are quite substantial, with a significant gain in height (1 to 2 inches) and a more normal appearing waistline. This confirms the work of Ascani (2), who noted that with reduction of the displacement by the hyperextension casting

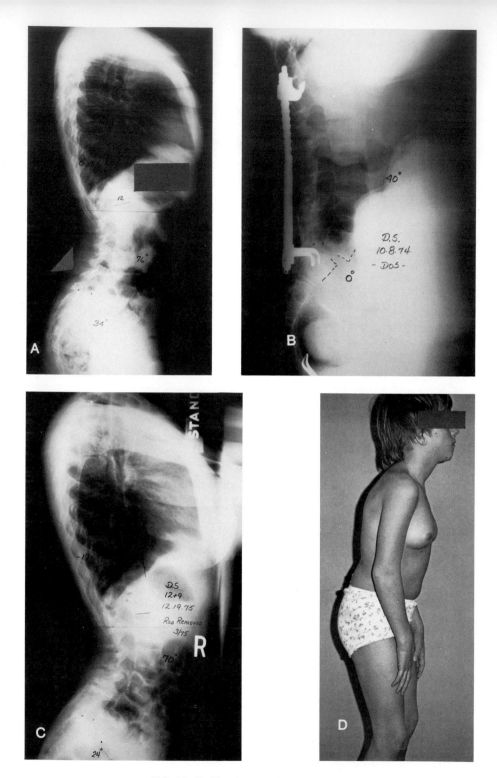

FIG. 9A–D. (*See legend facing page.*)

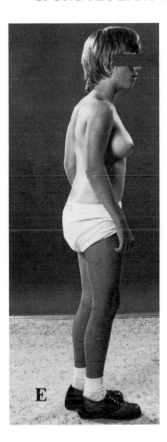

FIG. 9. Reduction of the spondylolisthesis is possible and may be carried out by the Harrington device **(A and B).** The rod is placed from T12 to sacrum but the fusion extends from L4 to sacrum. The rod is removed 1 year later **(C).** The initial appearance **(D)** and 2 year follow-up **(E).**

technique cases of partial paralysis and existing bowel and bladder disturbances disappeared (Fig. 11). One must consider that even with a spine fusion (without a Gill decompression) further slippage may continue to develop while the fusion is solidifying. This has been reported in 20 to 30% of patients with more advanced degrees of slippage (5,7,32). Therefore reduction and stabilization is an attractive alternative for these patients with slips greater than 50%. For slips less than 50%, the more standard techniques of fusion *in situ* would remain the treatment of choice.

Repair of the Defect

Techniques have also been described for direct repair of the defect in spondylolisthesis by either screw fixation across the fracture in the pars or fusion across the defect alone (6,27). These techniques may be valid for slippage of less than 25%, but for greater slippage they appear to be ineffective.

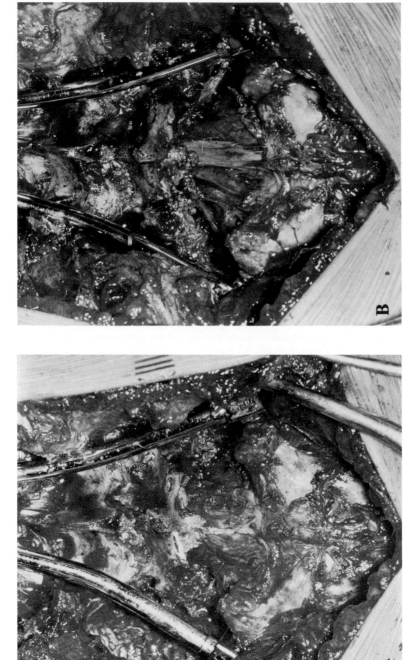

FIG. 10. Appearance of the dura and L5 roots before **(A)** and after **(B)** reduction. Before reduction the dura does not pulsate **(A)**, whereas afterward the root is visualized (L5) and the dura expends, fills out, and begins to pulsate **(B)**.

Anterior Interbody Fusion

Anterior interbody fusion for spondylolisthesis is seldom necessary in the child. Transperitoneal lumbar fusion was first performed by Capener in 1932 (11,17) and recently received increased attention as a method to be used in conjunction with posterior reduction of the spondylolisthesis and fusion (43). The reduction and the stability of reduction achieved by this technique appears greater than that achieved by posterior spine fusion with instrumentation by the Harrington technique. The exact indication for this method remains unclear, but it appears physiologically to be the most certain method of achieving an adequate reduction, a solid fusion, and prevention of further slippage. With the exposure, damage to the sacral plexus is a risk with resultant retrograde ejaculation in the male.

TREATMENT OF TRAUMATIC SPONDYLOLISTHESIS

Traumatic spondylolisthesis is generally managed successfully with plaster cast immobilization (37). Effective immobilization is best assured by the application of a cast which incorporates one thigh, facilitating increased immobilization of the lumbosacral articulation. It is of interest that some defects heal without treatment while the patient continues vigorous athletic activities (47). It is important to remember that acute fractures have medicolegal importance if it can be proved that the lesion was caused by a given injury or accident. This is extremely difficult, however, since pre injury x-rays are rarely available. If symptoms continue in spite of conservative management, operative intervention may be necessary, which consists of spinal stabilization by arthrodesis.

TREATMENT OF DEGENERATIVE SPONDYLOLISTHESIS

The treatment of degenerative spondylolisthesis (33,34,38) is basically that of the management of degenerative disc disease. Here, however, the situation is often complicated by spinal stenosis, which develops secondary to forward slippage, centrally placed facet joints, and exuberant bone formation from osteoarthritic spurring around the facets. Most of these patients can be treated by conservative management: analgesics, abdominal exercises, corsets, antiarthritic drugs, and reassurance. Conservative therapy is adequate in 90% of these patients (37). Neurologic symptoms secondary to spinal stenosis are what usually bring the patient to the doctor and which ultimately make surgical treatment necessary. Decompression is the procedure of choice (8). Myelography shows hourglass encroachment at the level of slipping and sometimes constriction sufficient enough to constitute a "block." A disc herniation at the level of slipping is also seen occasionally. The disc herniation may be at a level actually lower than the slippage. Surgery consists of a laminectomy using a posterior approach.

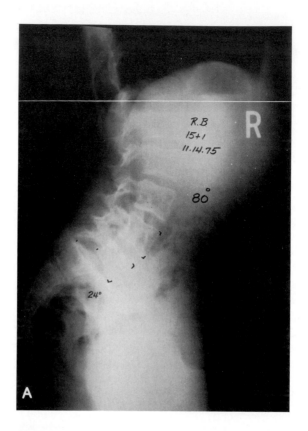

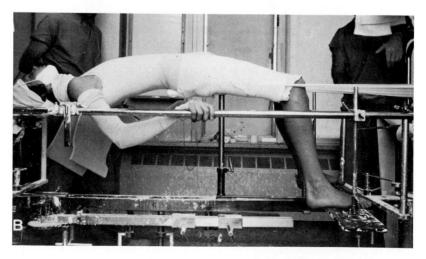

FIG. 11A–B. (See legend facing page.)

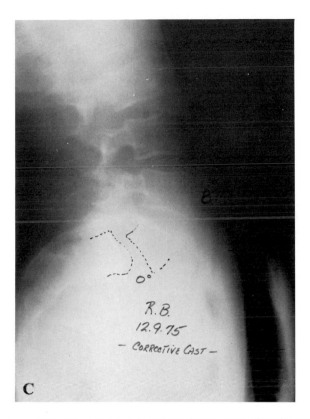

FIG. 11. The spondylolisthesis may be reduced by plaster, extending the sacrum and hips and applying longitudinal traction: Before **(A)** and after **(C)**.

The level at which the spinal canal is approached is sometimes difficult to identify because of transitional lumbosacral articulation or unsuspected fusion of the lumbosacral joints. Interoperative x-rays may be beneficial. The point of compression is where there is a slippage of L4 on L5 and the L5 nerve root becomes compressed as it passes between the upper edge of the body of L5 and the hypertrophic edge of the superior facet of the same vertebra (33). It is best, therefore, to remove part of the lamina of the vertebra above and below the level of slippage. The lateral recesses must be well decompressed so there is no question that the nerves are completely unroofed. If one confines the decompression to removing the lower half of the laminae and the spinous processes of the slipped vertebra, and the upper half of the laminae in the spinous process of the subadjacent vertebra, adequate decompression can usually be achieved without producing greater instability. The L5 root should be traced well out, taking off the corner of the superior articular process of L5 but usually not cutting through the pars of L5. Even after adequate decompression has been achieved, mobility of the dura may be impaired because of tethering of a nerve root which has become adherent to the underlying anulus. This should be carefully dissected off and Gelfoam used to prevent adherence of the soft tissues to the dura following decompression. The step-off due to the malalignment of the vertebral bodies at the level of the slip should be identified to confirm that the proper level has been decompressed. If a herniated disc is found, it should be removed. Occasionally the pars of L5 must be cut through in order to furnish adequate decompression, but this leads to greater instability with the possibility of further slippage. It is interesting, however, that this does not appear to make these patients symptomatically worse, and Rosenberg found that the increased slippage that may occur, which was as much as 15% during the year following surgery, did not subsequently progress, seeming to stabilize after that period (38). The question of whether spine fusion should be done is still controversial. It is our opinion that spine fusion is not necessary in patients older than age 60.

SCOLIOSIS AND SPONDYLOLISTHESIS

A long lumbar scoliosis or thoracolumbar scoliosis extending to the sacrum is often associated with spondylolisthesis and is secondary to lumbar muscle spasm. It usually remits with recumbency or relief of symptoms. It also may be expected to resolve following surgical stabilization of the spondylolisthesis. Occasionally, with delayed treatment, it may become structural and require treatment in its own right. If there is a coexisting thoracic idiopathic curvature, it should be managed as a separate problem. If it cannot be controlled with bracing or if it is too severe initially (greater than 45 to 50°), surgical correction of the curvature by spine fusion is indicated. If it is a double major curvature (i.e., a right thoracic and left lumbar curve), the problem becomes more complex since it may be necessary to extend the fusion from the upper thoracic spine all the way to the sacrum (i.e., treating the scoliosis as well as the spondylolisthesis together). The pseudarthrosis rate may be higher and the disability greater, secondary to such an extensive spine fusion. If there is a nonsymptomatic spondylolysis or a grade I spondylolisthesis at L5 to S1, the scoliosis fusion can extend down to L4 and the L4 to sacrum area can be left alone.

REFERENCES

1. Adkins, E. W. O. (1955): Spondylolisthesis. *J. Bone Joint Surg.*, 37B:48.
2. Ascani, C.: Personal communication.
3. Baker, D. R., and McHolick, W. (1956): Spondylolysis and spondylolisthesis in children. *J. Bone Joint Surg.*, 38A:933.
4. Borkow, S. E., and Kleiger, B. (1971): Spondylolisthesis in newborn: A case report. *Clin. Orthop.*, 81:71.
5. Bosworth, D. M., Fielding, J. W., Demarest, L., and Bonaquist, M. (1955): Spondylolisthesis. *J. Bone Joint Surg.*, 37A:707.

6. Buck, J. E. (1970): Direct repair of the defect in spondylolisthesis. *J. Bone Joint Surg.*, 52B:432.
7. Dandy, D. J., and Shannon, M. J. (1971): Lumbosacral subluxation. *J. Bone Joint Surg.*, 53B:578.
8. Davis, I. S., and Bailey, R. W. (1976): Spondylolisthesis: Indications for lumbar nerve root decompression and operative technique. *Clin. Orthop.*, 117:129.
9. Del Torto, U. (1965): The effect of transplants of patient arteries into the epiphysis of long bones. *Orthopaedic Research Society Annual Meeting*, New York.
10. Farfan, H. F., Osteria, V., and Lamy, C. (1976): The mechanical etiology of spondylolysis and spondylolisthesis. *Clin. Orthop.*, 117:40.
11. Freebody, D., Bendall, R., and Taylor, R. D. (1971): Anterior transperitoneal lumbar fusion. *J. Bone Joint Surg.*, 53B:617.
12. Gill, G. G., Manning, J. G., and White, H. L. (1955): Surgical treatment of spondylolisthesis without spine fusion. *J. Bone Joint Surg.*, 37A:493.
13. Harrington, P. R., and Dickson, J. H. (1976): Spinal instrumentation in the treatment of severe progressive spondylolisthesis. *Clin. Orthop.*, 117:157.
14. Harrington, P. R., and Tullos, H. S. (1971): Spondylolisthesis in children, observations and surgical treatment. *Clin. Orthop.*, 79:75.
15. Harris, R. I. (1951): Spondylolisthesis. *Ann. R. Coll. Surg. Engl.*, 8:259–297.
16. Herbiniaux, G. (1782): *Traite sur Divers Accouchemens Laborieux, et sur les Polypes de la Matrice*. Dehoubers, Bruxelles.
17. Hodgson, A. R., and Wong, S. K. (1968): A description of a technique and evaluation of results in anterior spinal fusion for deranged intervertebral disc and spondylolisthesis. *Clin. Orthop.*, 56:133.
18. Jackson, D. W., Wiltse, L. L., and Cirincione, R. J. (1976): Spondylolysis in the female gymnast. *Clin. Orthop.*, 117:68.
19. Kilian, H. F. (1854): *Schilderungen Neuer Beckenformen und Ihres Verhaltens in Leven, Mannheim*. Verlag von Bassermann & Mathy.
20. Lambl, W. (1858): *Beitrage zur Geburtskunde un Dynackologie, von F. W. v. Schanzoni*.
21. Lance, E. M. (1966): Treatment of severe spondylolisthesis with neural involvement, a report of two cases. *J. Bone Joint Surg.*, 48:883.
22. Laurent, L. E. (1958): Spondylolisthesis. *Acta Orthop. Scand. (Suppl.)*, 35.
23. Laurent, L. E., and Osterman, K. (1976): Operative treatment in spondylolisthesis in young patients. *Clin. Orthop.*, 117:85.
24. Lowe, R. W., Hayes, T. D., Kaye, J., Bagg, R. J., and Leukens, C. A. (1976): Standing roentgenograms in spondylolisthesis. *Clin. Orthop.*, 117:85.
25. Meyerding, H. W. (1932): Spondylolisthesis. *Surg. Gynecol. Obstet.*, 54:371–377.
26. Mosimann, P. (1961): Die histologie der spondylolyse. *Arch. Orthop. Unfallchir.*, 53:264.
27. Nachemson, A. (1976): Repair of the spondylolisthetic defect and intertransverse fusion for young patients. *Clin. Orthop.*, 117:101.
28. Nachemson, A., and Wiltse, L. L. (1976): Editorial comment: Spondylolisthesis. *Clin. Orthop.*, 117:2.
29. Neugebauer, F. L. (1976): The classic: A new contribution to the history and etiology of spondylolisthesis. *Clin. Orthop.*, 117:4.
30. Newman, P. H. (1965): A clinical syndrome associated with severe lumbosacral subluxation. *J. Bone Joint Surg.*, 47B:472.
31. Newman, P. H., and Stone, K. H. (1963): The etiology of spondylolisthesis, with a special investigation. *J. Bone Joint Surg.*, 45B:39.
32. Newman, P. H. (1973): Surgical treatment for derangement of the lumbar spine. *J. Bone Joint Surg.*, 55B:7.
33. Newman, P. H. (1976): Surgical treatment for spondylolisthesis in the adult. *Clin. Orthop.*, 117:106.
34. Osterman, K., Lindholm, T. S., and Laurent, L. E. (1976): Late results of removal of the loose posterior (Gill's operation) in the treatment of lytic lumbar spondylolisthesis. *Clin. Orthop.*, 117:121.
35. Phalen, G. S., and Dickson, J. A. (1961): Spondylolisthesis and tight hamstrings. *J. Bone Joint Surg.*, 43A:505.
36. Robert: (1855): *Monatsschr. Geburt. Frauenkrankh.*, 5:81.

37. Roche, M. B. (1950): Healing of bilateral fracture of the pars interarticularis of a lumbar neural arch. *J. Bone Joint Surg.*, 32A:428.
38. Rosenberg, N. J. (1976): Degenerative spondylolisthesis. *Clin. Orthop.*, 117:112.
39. Scaglietti, O., Frontino, G., and Bartolozzi, P. (1976): Technique of anatomical reduction of lumbar spondylolisthesis and its surgical stabilization. *Clin. Orthop.*, 117:164.
40. Scaglietti, O., Frontino, G., and Bartolozzi, P. (1970): Tecnica della ridozione de-la spondelolistesi lombare e sua contenzione definitive. *Atti Soc. Ital. O. T.*, 292–1970.
41. Snijder, J. G. N., Seroo, J. M., Snijer, C. J., and Schifvens, A. W. M. (1976): Therapy of spondylolisthesis by repositioning and fixation of the olisthetic vertebra. *Clin. Orthop.*, 117:149.
42. Stewart, T. D. (1953): The age incidence of neural arch defects in Alaskan natives, considered from the standpoint of etiology. *J. Bone Joint Surg.*, 35A:937.
43. Taddonio, R. F., and DeWald, F. L. (1976): Reduction and fusion of severe spondylolisthesis. Presented at the 11th Annual Scoliosis Research Society Meeting, Ottawa, Ontario.
44. Taillard, W. (1954): Le spondylolisthesis chez l'enfant et l'adolescent. *Acta Orthop. Scand.*, 24:115.
45. Taillard, W. F. (1976): Etiology of spondylolisthesis. *Clin. Orthop.*, 117:30.
46. Wiltse, L. L. (1962): The etiology of spondylolisthesis. *J. Bone Joint Surg.*, 44A:539.
47. Wiltse, L. L., and Jackson, D. W. (1976): Treatment of spondylolisthesis and spondylolysis in children. *Clin. Orthop.*, 117:92.
48. Wiltse, L. L., Newman, P. H., and MacNab, I. (1976): Classification of spondylolisthesis. *Clin. Orthop.*, 117:23.
49. Wiltse, L. L., Widell, E. H., and Jackson, D. W. (1975): Fatigue fracture: The basic lesion in intrinsic spondylolisthesis. *J. Bone Joint Surg.*, 57A:17.

Spinal Deformities and Neurological Dysfunction, edited by S. N. Chou and E. L. Seljeskog. Raven Press, New York © 1978.

Treatment of Occult Spinal Dysraphic Abnormalities (Occult Spinal Dysraphisms)

Donald L. Erickson

Department of Neurosurgery, University of Minnesota Hospital, Minneapolis, Minnesota 55455

Dysraphic states may occur as overt lesions (e.g., myelomeningoceles) or in a variety of covert abnormalities (e.g., diastematomyelia or persistent dermal sinus). The complex series of changes in the embryonic development of the neural tube allow for a wide variety of congenital anomalies. Some of these lesions may remain asymptomatic throughout life, whereas others produce disastrous and disabling neurologic problems. Neurosurgeons as well as orthopedic surgeons who deal with congenital spinal deformities must be keenly aware of the possible occult lesions responsible for neurologic deficit or congenital scoliosis. We have elected to discuss persistent dermal sinus and diastematomyelia in this chapter, although other defects such as lipoma of the cauda equina and tight filum terminale could probably fit into this grouping as well.

Diastematomyelia is rare, and, in our experience, persistent dermal sinus is even rarer. It is the presence of a large scoliosis center associated with our institution that accounts for the relative frequency with which we deal with these defects. Winter et al, in reviewing 392 patients with congenital scoliosis, found a 4.9% incidence of diastematomyelia (13). Not all of the patients in the series had myelograms, so presumably some of the defects went undetected. The associated clinical findings (discussed below) are now so well recognized it is less likely that future lesions will be missed.

The embryologic development of these lesions is not fully understood. Persistent dermal sinus appears to be due to a simple failure of appropriate separation of the neuroectoderm from the epithelial ectoderm with varying degrees of mesodermal maldevelopment (8). This leaves a persistent epithelium lined tract, which can penetrate as far as the center of the spinal cord. The mechanism of development is diastematomyelia is less clear (2,10). The diastasis of the spinal cord seems to be the primary defect which predisposes to the presence of a septum. The septum may then become calcified into the classic spur or remain simply as a fibrous band, with or without the typical dural separation (Fig. 1). The mesodermal maldevelop-

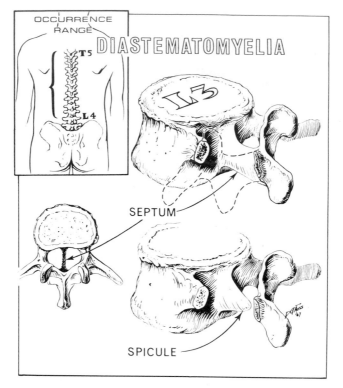

FIG. 1. Type and location of diastomatomyelic spur. (From ref. 7.)

ment, and hence the vertebral anomalies, is usually much more extensive in patients with diastematomyelia than it is in those with persistent dermal sinus.

RECOGNITION OF THE SYNDROME

A particular set of clinical findings occurs with sufficient frequency to indicate the diagnosis of an occult intraspinal defect. As already mentioned, some of these children may present with congenital scoliosis. Because only 5–10% of these children have associated intraspinal lesions, it would not be reasonable to subject all of them to myelography in order to make the diagnosis (13). Careful examination of the skin overlying the spine, particularly in the lumbar or lower thoracic area, discloses a hair patch, a port wine stain, a subcutaneous lipoma, or a small dimple in approximately 75% of the patients with one of these dysraphisms (3,6,7,13). Occurring with equal frequency in these children is a small leg and foot on one side (4,6,7). Although the latter abnormality is probably due to an underlying neurologic deficit, a specific sensory or reflex deficit in the extremity is found much less frequently. A number of these patients have sphincter disturbances, which is occasionally the presenting complaint.

There are some typical x-ray findings which are also frequently associated with the occult abnormalities (5,7,13). Most of the patients have spina bifida, although this may not be at the same level as the dyastematic spur or at the level of the dermal sinus. In nearly all patients with diastematomyelia there is an abnormal widening of the interpedicular distance at the level of the spur. Although perhaps not as common as widening, the presence of fusion and deformity of the posterior spinal elements have a very high association with the level of the diastematomyelic spur as noted by Hilal et al. (5). Tomography and even computerized tomography (12) of the spine may yield additional information, but the definitive test is myelography (5). The classic myelographic picture shows a split in the dye column as it surrounds the midline septum. In our experience, this has been apparent in the prone position but occasionally the septum does not reach the anterior aspect of the canal and a supine myelogram must be used to demonstrate the defect. Persistent dermal sinus is not so easily diagnosed myelographically, and if the tract is very thin or does not penetrate the spinal cord the myelogram may be normal.

RATIONALE FOR TREATMENT

In persistent dermal sinus the rationale for treatment is obvious. The risk of meningitis has been emphasized (8). The occurrence of repeated meningitis, particularly with coliform bacteria, should stimulate a search for the sometimes small, not so obvious skin lesion. The presence of this lesion even without neurologic deficit or spinal deformity demands total resection. If fusion of an associated spinal deformity is contemplated, it is our policy to resect the sinus tract initially and wait for wound healing, undertaking fusion at a second operation. The risk of fusion in the face of a contaminated defect is unwarranted. Also, if the defect persists cephalad into the spinal cord, removal of the sinus tract alone may be a time-consuming operation, requiring an extensive laminectomy. We believe it is unwise to perform an elective fusion in the presence of a fresh extensive laminectomy. The risk of postoperative complications (e.g., extradural hematoma) are much reduced if the initial surgery is allowed to heal and form a fibrous barrier over the exposed dura.

The rationale for repair of diastematomyelia is not always as obvious. One must recognize that congenital neurologic abnormalities in the form of a small leg and foot probably represent the lack of development, or *in utero* damage of neural elements, rather than dysfunction due to the presence of a spur or persistent traction on the spinal cord (10). Additional evidence for the neural maldevelopment etiology is the frequent presence of a small leg associated with persistent dermal sinus, even when the sinus does not penetrate the spinal cord. Our experience agrees with that reported in the literature, being that these neurologic and developmental deficits do not improve following removal of the spur (4,11).

It is recognized, however, that secondary neurologic complications such as bowel and bladder disturbance or increased dysfunction of the lower extremities sometimes develop as the child matures. There is some controversy regarding the mechanism of the secondary neurologic deficits. An attractive theory is the concept of differential growth of spinal cord and spinal canal, producing a traction injury on the neural elements due to the midline spur. In view of the work by Barson, which demonstrated that the majority of differential growth is completed at the age of 2 months, this theory seems less tenable (1). There is, however, significant excursion of the spinal cord within the canal produced by neck flexion and extension which could produce repeated minor trauma at the septum site sufficient to account for the progressive deficit. Further evidence that the traction theory is untenable is supported by Guthkelch (4), who applied silver clips to the pia and adjacent dura and found no separation of the clips over a period of time. Regardless of the cause of the neurologic deficits, the spur should be removed at the first sign of increasing neurologic problem because these neurologic deficits have been reversed by early surgical intervention (4).

It has been our policy to remove the spur in anyone who will be undergoing corrective surgery for spinal deformity. The primary reason for this has been the occasional sudden occurrence of severe neurologic deficit with manipulation of the spine in the presence of a diastematomyelic spur or any other intraspinal defect that prevents normal excursion of the spinal cord. Secondly, and of lesser importance, is the fact that an extensive fusion encompassing the site of the diastematomyelic spur would certainly complicate spur removal should the need arise later.

TECHNIQUES OF REPAIR

Matson emphasized the importance of being prepared to do an extensive laminectomy when one attempts removal of a persistent dermal sinus (8). Occasionally the tract turns cephalad for several segments before penetrating the dura or indeed penetrates the dura and then attaches to the spinal cord still some distance cephalad from the skin lesion. In our experience, however, the lesion typically ends at the dura one or two segments above the skin dimple. The operation should therefore be performed in a manner that allows extensive exposure, if necessary, but utilizing a minimum incision and bone resection to remove the entire tract adequately if it ends abruptly at the dural level. If the myelogram is normal and the tract narrows to a fibrous attachment at the dural surface, it is our policy not to open the dura and explore intradural contents. However, if there is an intraspinal defect on the myelogram, it is necessary to explore that as well, and adequately excise it if it is a continuation of the dermal sinus. It is possible to have multiple lesions, and we have seen patients with a myelomeningocele at one level and dermal sinus or diastematomyelia at another (4,5). If a subsequent fusion is contemplated, it is advantageous to do as little bone removal as possible, both in width and cephalocaudal direction. With magnification and micro instruments, it is unnecessary to have an extensive laminectomy to remove these lesions adequately.

The method described by Meacham for removal of the diastematomyelic spur has become our accepted technique (9). Once again, we remove a minimum of bone; it is generally unnecessary to remove any more than the lamina directly associated with the spur. Unlike intraspinal mass lesions,

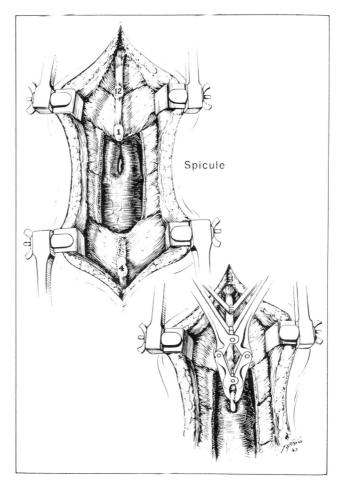

FIG. 2. Extradural removal at spur. (From ref. 7.)

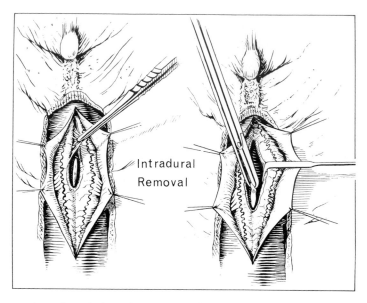

Intradural
Removal

FIG. 3. Completion of spur removal, intradural. (From ref. 7.)

where one must be careful to open the spine in a normal area first, we have found it safe to do a single level laminectomy at the spur site. As the last portion of lamina is being removed a small, sharp rongeurs is required so that one must be careful not to twist or dislodge the spur which sometimes has a small anterior attachment. Once the spur is exposed it can be cautiously removed piecemeal prior to opening the dura (Fig. 2). It is sometimes difficult to remove the most anterior portion of the spur completely until the dura is open (Fig. 3). Bipolar cautery is extremely helpful for the venous bleeding that often accompanies removal of the spur, especially at its anterior portion. Although it is unnecessary to close the anterior dura, this is occasionally the simplest way to control bleeding in that area, when bipolar cautery is not effective. There are usually numerous fine arachnoidal adhesions on the underside of the spinal cord, particularly where the diastematomyelia again becomes a single cord. These should be cut with a fine microscissors.

I generally discourage attempts at simultaneous lesion removal and fusion. By the very nature of fusion, which requires raw bone surfaces, hemostatis cannot be adequately obtained. Suction drainage is inappropriate because of the dural repair and risk of promoting a cerebrospinal fluid fistula. Anything but immaculate hemostasis in the face of a laminectomy, particularly after the dura has been opened, holds the risk of epidural hematoma and spinal cord injury. Because this is elective surgery it seems unreasonable to take any added risk in these children.

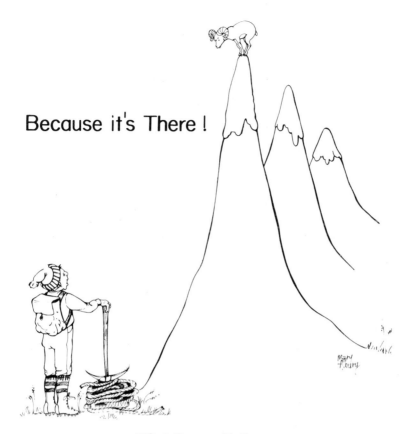

FIG. 4. Because it's there.

RESULTS

We have had no postoperative increase in neurologic deficit in our series of 12 patients with dermal sinus or diastematomyelia. They were all treated prior to any evidence of progressive neurologic complications, and there was no change observed in the pre-existing neurologic deficits. In one patient, back pain was the primary symptom, and that resolved following correction of the diastematomyelia. Because our experience has been favorable, we now recommend removal of any diastematomyelic spur encountered during infancy or childhood (Fig. 4). The presence of an asymptomatic spur in an adult hardly justifies removal.

SUMMARY

Occult intraspinal lesions (e.g., persistent dermal sinus or diastematomyelia) are rare and fascinating congenital anomalies. The clinical clues to their presence are midline dorsal skin lesions, neurologic deficits, hypoplastic extremities, or congenital scoliosis. The classic spine x-ray findings can be supported by myelography in establishing the diagnosis of these lesions. Surgical removal is recommended in persistent dermal sinus, primarily to prevent the occurrence of meningitis. It is our recommendation that the diastematomyelia be operated on during infancy or early childhood to prevent the development of subsequent neurologic deficits which may be associated either with maturation or surgical correction of the associated scoliosis.

REFERENCES

1. Barson, A. J. (1970): The vertebral level of termination of the spinal cord during normal and abnormal development. *J. Anat.*, 106:489.
2. Bremer, J. L. (1952): Dorsal intestinal fistula; accessory neurenterice canal; diastematomyelia. *Arch. Pathol.*, 54:132–138.
3. Burrows, F. G. O. (1968): Some aspects of occult spinal dysraphism: A study of 90 cases. *Br. J. Radiol.*, 41:496–507.
4. Guthketch, A. N. (1974): Diastematomyelia with median septum. *Brain*, 97:729–742.
5. Hilal, S. K., Marton, D., and Pollack E. (1974): Diastematomyelia in children. *Radiology*, 112:609–621.
6. James, C. C. M., and Lassman, L. P. (1964): Diastematomyelia, a critical survey of 24 cases submitted to laminectomy. *Arch. Dis. Child.*, 39:125–130.
7. Keim, H. A., and Greene, A. F. (1963): Diastamatomyelia and scoliosis. *J. Bone Joint Surg.*, 55:1425–1435.
8. Matson, D. D. (1969): *Neurosurgery of Infancy and Childhood.* Charles C Thomas, Springfield, Ill.
9. Meacham, W. F. (1967): Surgical treatment of diastematomyelia. *J. Neurosurg.*, 28:78–86.
10. Rokos, J. (1975): Pathogenesis of diastematomyelia and spina bifida. *J. Pathol.*, 117:155–161.
11. Shaw, J. F. (1975): Diastematomyelia. *Dev. Med. Child Neurol.*, 3:361–364.
12. Weinstein, M. A., Rothner, A. D., Duchesneau, P., and Bohn, D. F. (1975): Computer tomography in diastematomyelia. *Radiology*, 117:609–611.
13. Winter, R. B., Haven, J. J., Moe, J. H., and Lagaard, S. N. (1974): Diastematomyelia and congenital spine deformities. *J. Bone Joint Surg.*, 56-A:27–39.

Spinal Deformi
Dysfunction, edi
E. L. Seljeskog.
© 1978.

Treatment of Scoliosis and Possib Neurologic Complications

Robert B. Winter

Department of Orthopedic Surgery, University of Minnesota,
Minneapolis, Minnesota 55455

Neurologic dysfunction is the most feared complication following scoliosis surgery. Indeed, complete paraplegia is regarded by many as a fate worse than death. Unfortunately, cases of paralysis, both major and minor, are reported each year. As the methods for treatment have become more powerful, the number of neurologic lesions has risen, rather than fallen. Orthopedic surgeons treating major spine deformities must be cognizant of these problems and do their utmost to minimize them. Neurosurgeons may be called in to evaluate such patients and thus should also be aware of the nature of these problems.

CLASSIFICATION OF NEUROLOGIC COMPLICATIONS

Neurologic complications can be classified according to the following:

A. Lesions related to direct trauma
B. Lesions related to preoperative and postoperative traction
    1. Nerve roots
    2. Spinal cord
C. Lesions related to intraoperative traction by instrumentation
    1. Immediate onset
    2. Delayed onset
D. Miscellaneous
    1. Harrington hook erosion
    2. Dwyer screw insertion
    3. Root edema

REVIEW OF THE LITERATURE

Prior to 1950 there were few reports of neurologic problems related to scoliosis surgery. This was due to two factors, the first being the very few scoliosis operations being done, and second the very limited techniques available to the surgeon. Spine fusion was done without instrumentation and correction accomplished externally by casts with skin tolerance safely limiting the amount of spinal stretch.

In 1958 Risser and Norquist (7) reported three cases of paraplegia following routine cases of posterior spine fusion without instrumentation and without direct cord trauma. These three cases are of interest because the patients all had severe kyphosis, two being neurofibromatosis and one Morquio's disease. The cord was already stretched over the apex of the kyphosis and apparently the circulatory alteration (edema) of a posterior spine fusion was enough to tip the balance even though the cord was neither stretched nor directly traumatized.

It was not, however, until after 1960 that major concern arose about posttreatment paralysis. This was undoubtedly due to the introduction of powerful stretching devices, both internal and external. Harrington rods made their appearance around 1960, halofemoral traction in 1963, and the halohoop in 1968.

Moe (3) and Pinto (4) published articles on the complications related to scoliosis surgery. Among the many complications discussed have been the neurologic problems, both minor and major.

Ransford and Manning (6), in a major paper on the use of the halopelvic device ("halohoop"), described a disturbingly high percentage of neurologic problems. Of 118 patients placed in the halopelvic device, there were six with abducens palsies, five with hypoglossal palsies, two with glossopharyngeal palsies, six with brachial plexus palsies, four with sciatic palsy, and two with paraplegia, one permanent (diastematomyelia) and one recovering. All the paralysis problems, both root and cord, occurred in the first 62 patients in whom solid distraction rods were used. The second group of 56 patients had spring-loaded rods. This group had no neurologic problems.

Wilkins and MacEwen (9) reported on 59 patients undergoing halofemoral traction; seven in halopelvic and four in halo casts. Six had cranial nerve dysfunction, the 6th cranial nerve being the most frequently involved. Also noted was a combined 9th, 10th, and 12th cranial nerve palsy with difficulty in speech, swallowing, and respiration. All six patients had prompt relief of their symptoms by release of the traction.

Winter (10) reported a patient with simultaneous anterior and posterior wedge osteotomy who developed paraplegia 72 hr later. This case was complicated by severe congenital kyphosis, and the patient was in halofemoral traction during and following osteotomy (Fig 3).

The Scoliosis Research Society was founded in 1966, with one of its immediate projects being the formation of morbidity and mortality committees. It has been the yearly monitoring and reporting by the morbidity committee, summarized by MacEwen in 1975 (2), that led to the greatest understanding of these catastrophic complications.

There have been 87 patients reported with neurologic complications following scoliosis surgery (7,885 cases). This represents an incidence of 0.72%. Of the 87, 74 had major cord lesions, half, complete paraplegia and half incomplete; 36% recovered completely, 32% had partial recovery, and 32% had no recovery. Of the 74 major cord lesions, 42 were related to Harrington instrumentation and fusion, 20 occurred in posterior fusion without instrumentation, and 6 of the patients became paraplegic following skeletal traction.

A relatively high number of patients with congenital scoliosis appeared in this series. Thirty-two percent of the reported problems were associated with congenital spine deformities, although the general frequency of congenital scoliosis is only 10%. Idiopathic scoliosis constitutes over 85% of cases of scoliosis in most series, but only 43% of the complications in this study occurred in patients with idiopathic scoliosis.

Of the 42 patients with paraplegia following Harrington rod insertion, 26 had the rods removed postoperatively. Of the 24 patients with complete paralysis, 12 made a good or excellent recovery and 12 made no recovery. All 18 patients with incomplete paralysis made a good or excellent recovery.

Of the 12 patients whose rods were removed less than 3 hr after the paraplegia was noted, 9 made a complete recovery. Of the 14 who had rod removal later than 3 hr after the paraplegia was noted, only 8 made a complete recovery, and 7 of the 8 had incomplete paralysis. Of the 16 patients who did not have their rods removed, only 5 made a complete recovery.

This report clearly indicates certain patients are "at risk" for paraplegia. The high-risk groups are: (a) congenital spine deformity regardless of the magnitude of the curve, and (b) severe curves, i.e., those above 90°.

Those with congenital curves seem to be at high risk because of the high frequency of tethered spinal cords. This tethering may be a relatively obvious diastematomyelia or a quite obscure fibrous band or low-lying conus.

The highest-risk patient is the one with thoracic congenital kyphosis, especially if the kyphosis is sharp and angular, is a "pure" kyphosis (no scoliosis), and is centered at the "watershed" area of T4 to T9. One is tempted to say that such a patient should not have spine fusion because of this high risk. However, this is the patient who will undoubtedly develop spontaneous paraplegia if not fused.

In the other high-risk group is the patient with a "big" curve (i.e., above 90°), especially if the curve is rigid and the patient an adult. Such patients represent failures of the medical profession, since, as a generality, no one should be allowed to develop a 90°+ curve. *Preventing* the condition that produces a high-risk patient by adequate brace treatment and earlier fusion is the best answer to this problem.

CLINICAL MANIFESTATIONS AND MANAGEMENT

Lesions Related to Direct Trauma

Although the most obvious of all neurologic lesions, the lesion produced by direct trauma is probably the least common. Direct trauma results from direct contact of an instrument with the spinal cord. This can be a periosteal elevator, curet, or gouge. It is probably most common with a periosteal elevator, the surgeon unsuspectingly falling into the spinal canal while exposing the spine, usually because of an unsuspected spina bifida.

This has occurred only once in the author's personal experience. In this particular instance, a routine posterior exposure was being made of a previously fused spine with loss of correction due to a suspected pseudarthrosis. The periosteal elevator plunged into the spinal canal in an area where the previous fusion had been eroded away by a dural cyst due to neurofibromatosis. The dura was not penetrated. The patient awoke from surgery with total motor and sensory paralysis of the left leg plus a bladder paralysis. Her bladder recovered within 10 days, and the leg began to recover at 14 days. Complete recovery required 6 months.

The worst such incidence was a patient operated elsewhere and sent to the author 4 years later for further surgery. In the original operation, a diastematomyelia had not been appreciated, and at exposure the very abnormal bony anatomy led to the exposure of some "peculiar" white tissue (one-half of the spinal cord), which was biopsied. This resulted in permanent paralysis of one leg.

This above problem resulted from the attempts of an orthopedic surgeon to do scoliosis surgery without a single previous experience at such a major procedure. The diastematomyelia was readily apparent even on the plain x-rays taken before surgery. The patient should have been referred to a scoliosis center for treatment.

Lesions Related to Preoperative and Postoperative Traction Devices

Skeletal traction has become quite common in the correction of severe curvatures. It has become justifiably popular since it permits slow, cautious correction of truly terrible spine deformities. Patients whose pulmonary functions were so severely impaired as to be totally inoperable have been marvelously improved by such traction and have been thus converted to safe operative risks.

Such traction, however, is a two-edged sword. Strong skeletal traction, usually by a halo plus some form of countertraction at the pelvis, femors, or tibias, not only stretches the axial skeleton but also the spinal cord and the nerves exiting from the cord.

The stronger the traction, the more likely is complication. The most powerful traction device is the halohoop, but this device also produces the highest percentage of neurologic complications.

Neurologic damage can occur during the phase of preoperative traction or even after fusion while in some type of traction device. Either the cord or peripheral nerves may be involved.

The cranial nerves are often the first affected, most commonly the 6th cranial nerve (abducens). Other cranial nerves involved have been the 9th, 10th, and 12th. The brachial plexus has also been involved but seldom the sacral plexus. The bladder frequently shows the first sign of neurologic dysfunction, with inability to void due to a flaccid bladder.

Such peripheral nerve lesions and bladder problems should be detected promptly by daily neurologic examinations, and they usually respond promptly to reduction of traction or elimination of the traction weights altogether. In practical experience, total elimination of weights has not always been necessary. After several days of normal neurologic function, the weights can slowly and carefully be reapplied, often without producing neurologic complications, even at weights beyond the original level that produced the neurologic deficits.

One male child seen by the author had a severe cervicothoracic scoliosis due to neurofibromatosis. He developed a brachial plexus palsy with 4 kg of traction on a halo. The weights were reduced to 2 kg and the palsy disappeared within 24 hr. The weights were gradually resumed and finally reached 15 kg without neurologic troubles. Ten kilograms is now our maximal traction on a halo.

Despite these successes, other patients have been unable to tolerate weights beyond a certain level regardless of the slowness or cautiousness of application.

The treatment of such complications is obviously the prompt removal of traction. If removed within a few hours of development of the complication, the results are almost universally satisfactory. Administration of steroids, exploration, and other procedures have not been necessary.

Spinal cord lesions related to traction are more ominous than nerve root lesions. Most of the severe problems are related to instrumentation, but a few have been reported due to pre- or postoperative traction.

The usual problem is the patient with a congenital kyphosis. The spinal cord is already "at risk," having been angulated over the apex of the kyphosis. In many such cases, the cord is probably also "tethered" caudally and thus lacks normal "stretchability." With the addition of longitudinal traction, the cord is pulled against the apex of the kyphosis, probably compromising its precarious blood supply. This is most frequently seen with sharp, angular kyphoses at the "watershed" region of T4 to T9.

Four such lesions have been seen at our center during the past 10 years. Three patients had congenital kyphosis and one severe kyphoscoliosis due to diastrophic dwarfism. All four patients had halofemoral traction prior to surgery *without* neurologic problems. Two awoke from surgery with complete paraplegia (anterior spinal artery syndrome) and never recovered. One developed paraplegia 72 hr postoperatively and eventually recovered (Fig. 3), and the third developed paraplegia 5 days after posterior fusion and never recovered, dying of urinary tract infection 2 years later.

In such cases, it appears that the stretched cord is "at risk," and the edema

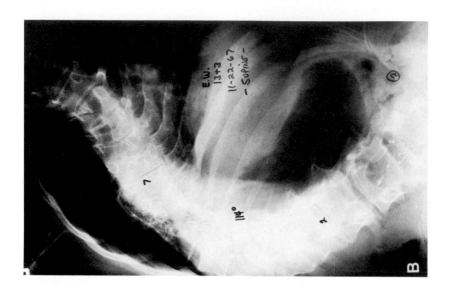

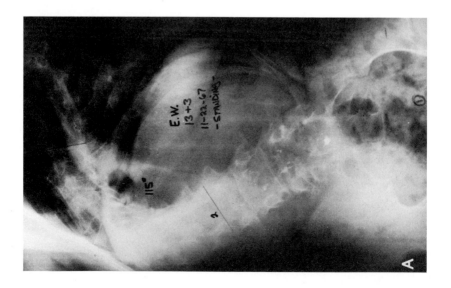

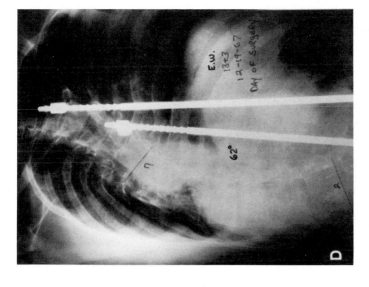

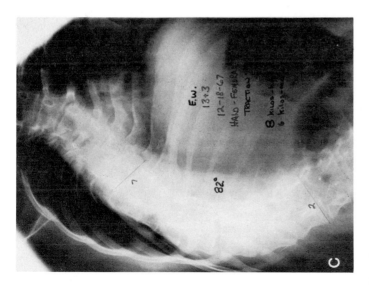

FIG. 1. E.W. **A:** This is a 13-year-old female with congenital scoliosis, cavus feet, and a low thoracic hair patch. Her curve is 115° standing and has been rapidly progressive. **B:** Supine position. Her curve is 114°, indicating severe rigidity. Anomalous vertebrae are noted in the midthoracic spine and at the lumbosacral level. A myelogram had been done 1 year previously (elsewhere) and was read as negative. A new myelogram was repeated and was again "normal." **C:** Halofemoral traction with 8 kg of traction on the skull and 6 kg on each femur. The curve was improved to 82°. Traction weights of more than this resulted in inability to void. **D:** On the day of surgery in which a spine fusion from T2 to S1 was done, two Harrington rods were also added, correcting the curve to 62°. She was neurologically normal immediately postoperatively but 4 hr later, had become almost completely paraplegic. The rods were removed promptly, and she made a good but not perfect recovery.

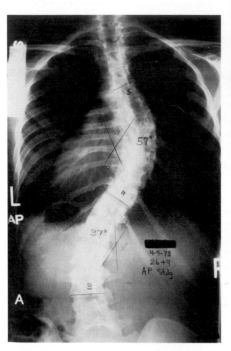

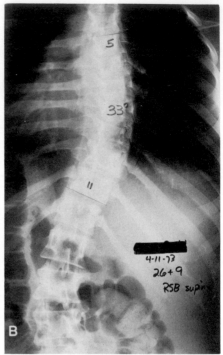

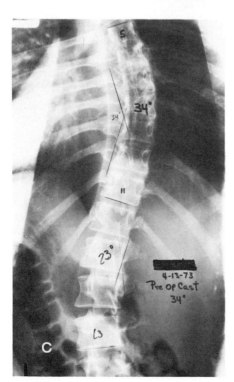

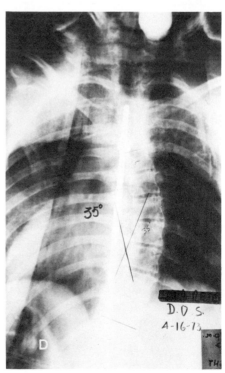

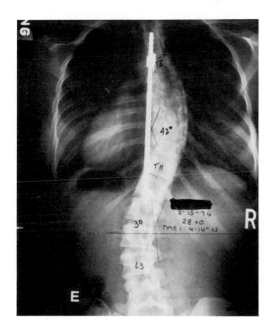

E

FIG. 2. E.R. **A:** This 26-year-old female was seen for progressive and painful 57° thoracic scoliosis. The neurologic examination was normal. **B:** A bending film revealed easy correctibility to 33°. **C:** She was placed in a preoperative cast, giving correction to 34°. **D:** Correction in surgery to 35° with a Harrington rod. Prior to taking this x-ray and immediately following rod insertion, the "wake-up test" had been done. She was completely unable to move her legs or feet although she could clench her fists on command. The rods were reduced in tension by one ratchet of the rod (5 mm), and she immediately awoke from surgery with no neurologic deficit and no recollection of the "wake-up test." **E:** At 19 months postoperation her curve is reasonably corrected and solidly fused. She has remained neurologically negative.

or circulatory changes associated with surgery tip the balance. The patient awaking from surgery with complete paralysis has a poor prognosis for recovery, whereas the lesion that develops while the patient is in traction before or after surgery has a good prognosis if it is recognized early and the weights removed promptly.

The two earliest signs of cord problems in traction are urinary bladder retention and a "heavy feeling" in the thighs. These occur a few hours prior to complete paralysis.

Lesions Related to Intraoperative Distraction (Harrington Rods)

Harrington rods have been one of the most important of all advances in the treatment of spinal deformities. Patients who previously had to spend 6 months in bed and a year in a cast are now routinely ambulated at 7 days, home in 12 days, back to school in 18 days, and out of their casts in 9 months. With such blessings have also come problems, and the worst of these is paraplegia (Fig. 1).

Harrington rods can cause paraplegia. This is a problem of stretching the spinal cord and its blood supply. It is unknown whether the specific lesion is inside the cord or outside, but the result is the same. Furthermore, if the patient awakes from the anesthetic with complete paraplegia, the likelihood of recovery is very small, even with immediate rod removal.

This catastrophic complication haunts all scoliosis surgeons and is the most feared of all complications. What can be done about it? A few surgeons have chosen not to use rods, performing only a fusion and using cast correction. This solves the problem in patients with the less severe curves, but these patients virtually never experience paralysis anyway.

Other surgeons continue to use rods but simply do not stretch the spine very much; they thus achieve less correction but at much less risk. This is also a good choice, but it does not eliminate all risks since some patients cannot tolerate any stretch, even a slight one.

Finally, there is a group of scoliosis surgeons who use intraoperative neurologic monitoring to see if paralysis has been induced. As soon as the rod is inserted, the patient is partially awakened (to the point of being able to respond to verbal command, although there is total amnesia) and asked to move the feet. Being able to move the feet on command is positive proof of intact cord function. A deeper level of anesthesia is then resumed. This technique was developed in France by Stagnara and colleagues (1,8) and is commonly called the "Stagnara wake-up test" (Fig. 2).

We have been using this technique for 4 years, encompassing approximately 600 rod insertions. Four patients have had positive "wake-up" tests. In all four, lessening of the distraction by as little as 5 mm has resulted in immediate conversion of the "wake-up" test to normalcy. All four patients awoke from surgery without motor deficit and remained neurologically normal (Fig. 2).

In the future, we are hopeful that some sort of electronic neurologic monitoring (e.g., intraoperative evoked potential recording) can be applied during surgery to replace the relatively crude wake-up test.

There is a second type of paraplegia related to rod insertion. In this type, the patient awakes from surgery neurologically intact but develops paraplegia 4–72 hr later. The onset is gradual over several hours. When the paraplegia is detected, the patient must be returned to the operating room *immediately* and the rods removed.

This type of paralysis appears to be related to progressive hypoperfusion of the cord. Ponte (5) reported two cases in which blood transfusion to restore normal blood pressure resulted in complete correction of the paralysis.

Such cases of "late-onset" paralysis respond much differently from the intraoperative type. With rod removal within 4 hr of onset, total recovery is the rule. If the rods are not removed until 8 hr or more after the onset of paralysis, recovery seldom occurs. The treatment is prompt recognition and immediate rod removal. Laminectomy is not indicated. Steroids alone do not seem to help.

Certain patients have a high susceptibility to such rod paraplegia. This is particularly true of congenital spine deformities, especially when the cord is tethered by tight filum terminale, diastematomyelia, or other dysraphic

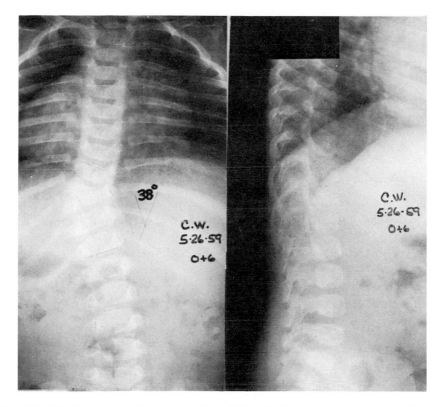

FIG. 3A. C.W. A 6-month-old female with a mild scoliosis due to a hemivertebra. There is no kyphosis.

condition (Fig. 3). In such patients we prefer not to use Harrington rods; and if used, the wake-up test must be done.

Other Instrumentation Problems

Harrington Hook Erosion

On rare occasions a Harrington hook can slowly erode through a lamina, resulting in pressure on a nerve root (usually in the lumbar spine). This may become manifest several years after the original procedure. Removal of the hook, exploration of the nerve root, and repair of the dura are indicated. In more than 2,000 rod insertions at this center, this has happened only three times.

Dwyer Procedure

The Dwyer procedure is a totally different concept of curve correction. Rather than lengthen the short side, it shortens the long side, thus avoiding

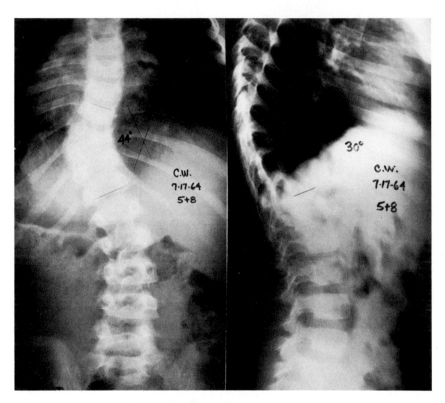

FIG. 3B. C.W., at age 5 years 8 months. The scoliosis was slightly worse, and a mild kyphosis had appeared. The potential hazards of this lesion were not appreciated by her physician and no treatment was given.

any stretching of the cord or nerve roots. When initially proposed, many feared paraplegia since five to nine segmental vessels are routinely ligated on one side. In practice, however, this proved to be no problem since no paraplegia has resulted from this procedure during the 10 years of its use.

One case of paraplegia resulted from inadvertent penetration of the spinal canal by a screw. Such incidents can be prevented only by secure knowledge of anatomy in the operating room. Since approximately 1,000 Dwyer procedures have been done throughout the world during the past 10 years, and an average of six screws are inserted in each case, only one misplacement among 6,000 insertions is acceptable.

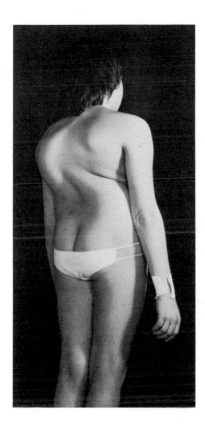

FIG. 3C. C.W., age 13, when she presented to the author. She was neurologically normal.

Root Edema

Many procedures involve dissection near or around nerve roots. This is necessary in order to identify and protect the root. Nevertheless, this dissection may itself result in irritation of the root with temporary, partial dysfunction. Such problems usually resolve spontaneously. If there is complete root paralysis, however, one should suspect the root is compressed by bone, and the patient should be explored and the root decompressed.

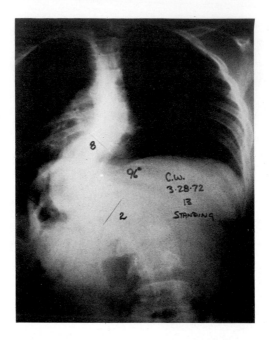

FIG. 3D. C.W., age 13, an AP x-ray showing a 96° scoliosis.

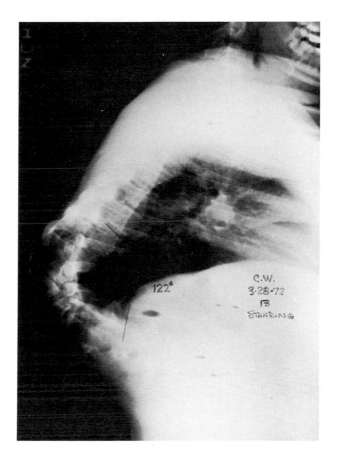

FIG. 3E. C.W., age 13, a lateral x-ray showing a 122° kyphosis.

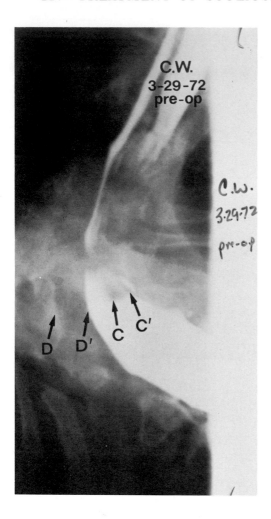

FIG. 3F. C.W., age 13, a preoperative myelogram showing displacement of the cord (c-c¹) to the concavity of the curve and displacement of the dura away from the bony canal on the convexity (d-d¹). There was no tethering or space-occupying lesion noted.

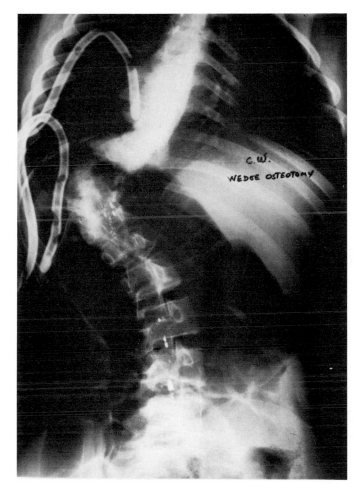

FIG. 3G. C.W.; an x-ray taken in halo-femoral traction in the P.A.R. following simultaneous anterior and posterior hemivertebra excision. She was neurologically normal until 60 hr postoperation when paralysis developed over a 12-hr period. The traction was removed and steroids were given, but the paraplegia became worse. She was returned to the operating room and the wound explored. No cause for the paralysis could be seen except that the cord was kinked over a kyphosis. She subsequently underwent a posterior fusion and compression instrumentation, and began to recover 8 weeks after the first operation. Full recovery required 16 months. An anterior fusion was subsequently done to correct a pseudoarthrosis.

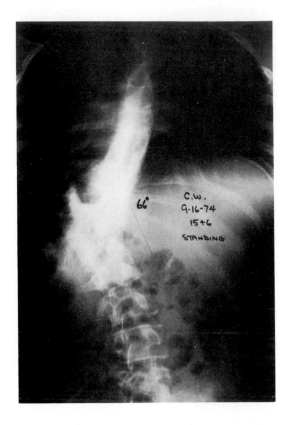

FIG. 3H. An AP x-ray 2 years later showing a scoliosis of 66° and a solid fusion.

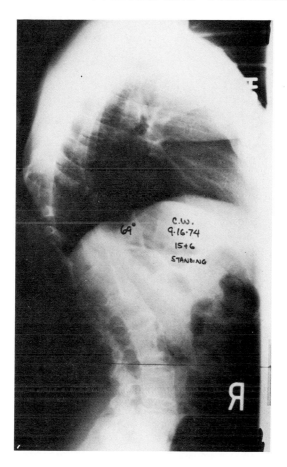

FIG. 31. A lateral x-ray at that time showing a kyphosis of 64° and a solid fusion.

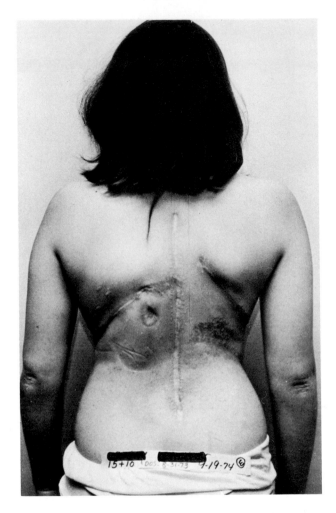

FIG. 3J. A posterior photograph at that time showing the corrected spine but multiple scars.

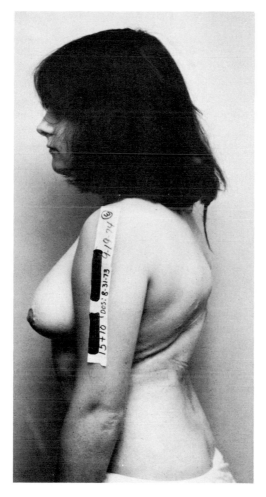

FIG. 3K. A lateral photograph to show the kyphotic correction.

SUMMARY

Neurologic complications of root and cord are a very real possibility in the surgical treatment of major spine deformity. The risks are not uniform; i.e., certain problems have a much higher risk rate than others. Proper identification of high-risk patients and careful clinical management of these cases by special techniques can result in many fewer neurologic complications.

Many problems arise from the necessity of treating large curves when the spine has reached a fairly rigid condition, thus necessitating rather strong corrective techniques. Earlier correction of such deformities, or even prevention by braces, prevents the need for drastic treatment modalities. Thus early identification of curves in children is critical.

Complications related to skeletal traction (e.g., halofemoral, halotibial, or halopelvic traction) are prevented by careful neurologic monitoring and prompt reduction of weights at the first sign of dysfunction.

Complications related to the intraoperative use of Harrington rods are prevented by judicious distraction, the use of intraoperative neurologic monitoring, the avoidance of rods in high-risk cases, and prompt rod removal if there is any evidence of neurologic compromise during the postoperative period.

Neurologic complications are the most feared in scoliosis surgery. They are better prevented than treated.

REFERENCES

1. Crawford, A. H., Jones, C. W., Perisho, J. A., and Herring, J. A. (1976): Hypnosis for monitoring intraoperative spinal cord function. *Anesth. Analg.,* 55:42–44.
2. MacEwen, G. D. (1975): Acute neurologic complications in the treatment of scoliosis (a report of the Scoliosis Research Society). *J. Bone Joint Surg.,* 57A:404–408.
3. Moe, J. H. (1967): Complications of scoliosis treatment. *Clin. Orthop.,* 53:21–30.
4. Pinto, W. C. (1973): Complications of surgical treatment of scoliosis. *Isr. J. Med. Sci.,* 9:837–842.
5. Ponte, A. (1974): Postoperative paraplegia due to hypercorrection of scoliosis and drop of blood pressure. *J. Bone Joint Surg.,* 56A:444.
6. Ransford, A. O., and Manning, C. W. S. F. (1975): Complications of halo-pelvic distraction for scoliosis. *J. Bone Joint Surg.,* 57B:131–137.
7. Risser, J. C., and Norquist, D. M. (1958): A followup study of the treatment of scoliosis. *J. Bone Joint Surg.,* 40A:555–569.
8. Vauzelle, C., Stagnara, P., and Jouvinroux, P. (1973): Functional monitoring of spinal cord activity during spinal surgery. *Clin. Orthop.,* 93:173–178.
9. Wilkins, C., and MacEwen, G. D. (1974): Halo-traction affecting cranial nerves. *J. Bone Joint Surg.,* 56A:1540.
10. Winter, R. B. (1976): Congenital kyphoscoliosis with paralysis following hemivertebra excision. *Clin. Orthop.,* 119:116–125.

Spinal Deformities and Neurological Dysfunction, edited by S. N. Chou and E. L. Seljeskog. Raven Press, New York © 1978.

External Fixation of the Spine

James M. Morris

Department of Orthopedic Surgery, University of California San Francisco, San Francisco, California 94143

The many types of external spinal appliances can be roughly divided into two types: (a) corrective and (b) supportive or "immobilizing." The corrective appliances include the Milwaukee and the Boston braces, used in treating scoliosis and kyphosis. Supportive or "immobilizing" supports or braces include a large variety of braces of different size designed to support the spine and restrict its motion in certain planes. This discussion is limited to the external support brace.

Differentiation should be made between support for acute traumatic instability of the spine and so-called chronic instability secondary to degenerative disc disease or pseudarthrosis of the spine after failed fusion. Acute instability, especially if there is a potential for neurological compromise, generally requires the use of halopelvic or halofemoral immobilization, or internal fixation and immobilization. This chapter deals with the problem of chronic instability, by far the most common condition for which external support is used, and which generally involves low back bracing for degenerative disc disease, failed spinal surgery, and complications of osteoporosis.

In the classic concept of bracing, the magnitude of the forces that the brace applies to the body varies with (a) the design of the brace or support and the tightness with which it is worn, and (b) the patient's attempt to move against the brace. Lusskin and Berger (2) pointed out that there are positive and negative physiological effects of bracing.

PHYSIOLOGICAL CONSEQUENCES OF LOW BACK BRACING

Positive Consequences

1. Increased intracavitary pressure provides trunk support and thereby decreases the demand on the abdominal and spinal musculature, ligaments, and intervertebral discs.

2. Restriction of motion provides relief of pain and decreases demands on the spinal elements.

3. Modification of skeletal alignment provides: (a) relief of pain by decreasing the weight on the diseased segments (extension produces weight transfer to the posterior elements and decreases weight on the vertebral bodies; and flexion produces weight transfer to the bodies and decreases the weight on the posterior elements); and (b) control of deformity, i.e., lordosis, kyphosis, and scoliosis.

Negative Consequences

1. Weakness follows reduced functional demand.
2. Muscular atrophy follows prolonged disuse.
3. Contracture follows immobilization and atrophy.
4. Bracing may produce psychological dependence and enhanced physical dependence.
5. Symptoms may increase after any of the above or with progressive disease, a wrongly prescribed brace, or a poorly fitted brace.

Brace and Support Designs

Over the years a large number of braces and supports have been designed and were named after the designer or locale. Supports in the past were largely prescribed on a regional basis, depending on the availability and the training of the orthotist. In an effort to standardize the terminology used to refer to the many supports, a New York University group proposed the following classifications:

Proposed NYU terminology	*Examples of common historical names*
Lumbosacral A-P control brace	chairback
Lumbosacral A-P and M-L control brace	Knight
Lumbosacral P and M-L control brace	Williams
Thoracolumbar A-P control brace	Taylor
Thoracolumbar and M-L control brace	Knight-Taylor
Thoracolumbar A-P, M-L, and rotary control brace	Cowhorn or Arnold
Thoracolumbar A control brace	Anterior hyperextension or Jewett

Such classifications are valuable in allowing more precise and standardized prescription writing. However, for purposes of this brief review of the mechanics of external spinal support, I prefer a simpler classification system.

Practical designation of spinal supports
Corrective (e.g., Milwaukee)
"Immobilizing" or supportive
   Long (Taylor and Arnold)
   Short (Knight, chairback, Williams)
Corsets

WHAT DOES A SUPPORT DO?

It has been widely recognized and demonstrated that braces and supports in current use cannot completely immobilize the spine. This is especially true in the lumbosacral region.

In the low back area, the region for which most supports are prescribed, bracing is a controversial matter. A variety of braces and other supports are available, but many practitioners shun the use of any support at all, citing the potential deleterious effects. However, if we accept the fact that a low back support can help alleviate symptoms in certain patients at certain times, it becomes valuable to outline a rationale to support their use. In order to do this we must know just what a brace or support can and cannot accomplish. It should be stressed at the outset that the use of the back support, except in rare cases, is a short-term or temporary measure only because prolonged usage may result in physiological dependence.

In 1957 Norton and Brown (4) studied the immobilizing capacity of back braces, paying particular attention to flexion and extension at the lumbosacral level. Kirschner wire markers were inserted into the spinous processes of appropriate lumbar vertebrae and into one of the posterior superior iliac spines. The change in angulation formed by adjacent wires demonstrated the motion occurring at the intervening interspace with and without external support (Fig. 1).

A wide variation of motion at the lower three intervertebral disc spaces was found in their subjects. There was a wide range of motion and variation in the rate of progression of flexion in the course of flexing the spine. Sitting was found to be associated with pronounced flexion of the lower two lumbar interspaces. In fact, flexion at the fourth lumbar interspace in the slump position was greater than when the same subject stood in maximum forward flexion. Norton and Brown stressed that the action of various back supports undoubtedly varied according to the lumbar flexion pattern of the individual, but they were unable to elaborate on this point.

Observations of the effects of a long back support (e.g., a Taylor or Arnold brace) during forward flexion and sitting indicated that the concentration of forces from the brace was located at or near the thoracolumbar junction and effectively restricted motion at this level. This concentration, however, was too high to immobilize the lower lumbar segments, and in fact

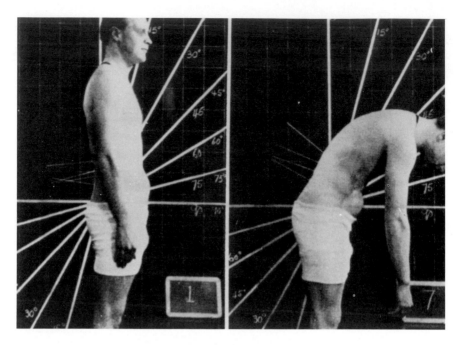

FIG. 1. Evaluation of posture and motion of the lumbosacral spine by means of percutaneous Steinmann pins. (From ref. 4.)

lumbosacral flexion was greater in some subjects when they wore a long brace than when they had no support (Fig. 2). None of the braces tested did more than limit interspace flexion. Actual immobilization never occurred. It was noted that the effect of most braces was to reduce the arc of motion in flexion, and in some cases the arc of motion was shifted toward the extension side of neutral; however, none of the supports studied demonstrate a clearly consistent pattern in all subjects.

Norton and Brown (4) stated that "it seems highly unlikely that any device applied to the exterior of the body can effectively splint the lumbosacral region." They pointed out that the effectiveness of the support, with respect to immobilization, seemed to be related more to the discomfort produced than to the magnitude of the force developed between the apparatus and the back. None of the supports they tested produced forces on the paraspinal musculature approaching an uncomfortable degree during slight forward bending. They stressed that a careful history would often determine whether flexion or extension of the lumbosacral area was more comfortable and the physician could then prescribe a suitable back support rather than rely on empirical application of a support.

Transverse rotation is a significant factor at the lumbosacral level, perhaps even more significant than flexion-extension. Because of the orientation of

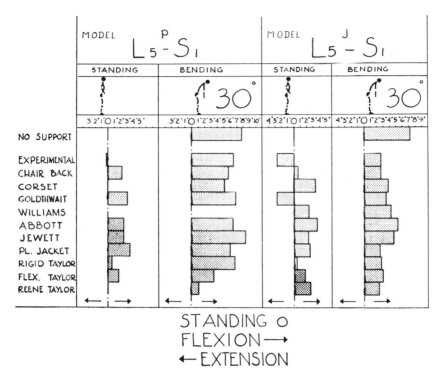

STANDING ○
FLEXION →
← EXTENSION

FIG. 2. Forward bend, two models. Effect of supports on the L5–S1 interspace. (From ref. 4.)

the posterior facets in the lumbar region, rotation produces shearing stresses on the anulus that may aggravate or accelerate degenerative changes. In contrast, the result of facet orientation in the thoracic spine is that the center of rotation lies at the center of the body, allowing easier rotation.

Lumsden and Morris (1) studied the effects of spinal supports on lumbosacral rotation. Pins were inserted into the spinous processes of the fifth lumbar vertebra and both posterior superior iliac spines in suitable subjects. A crossbar connected the two iliac crests, and rotation was measured by means of a relative rotation transducer connected to the pin in the L5 spinous process and the crossbar (Fig. 3). Using this transducer, only axial rotation in the transverse plane was recorded. An average of approximately 6° of rotation at the lumbosacral level was found during maximum rotation while the subject was standing. Approximately 1.5° of rotation occurred during normal walking. The amount of rotation at the lumbosacral level could not be correlated with such factors as body build, age, or as observed roentgenographically the orientation of the posterior facets (i.e., "tropism") or the height of the lumbosacral disc.

A modified chairback brace was relatively effective in restricting rotation

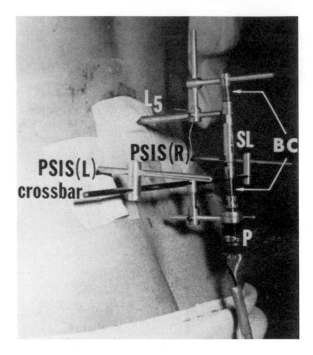

FIG. 3. Transducer affixed to pins and crossbar. L5 = pin in the spinous process of the fifth lumbar vertebra. PSIS (R) and PSIS (L) = pins in the posterior superior iliac spines, right and left, respectively. SL = slide mechanism allowing flexion and extension of the fifth lumbar vertebra. BC = bellows-type flexible coupling allowing bend in the vertical component of the slide. P = potentiometer with wires leading to the Visicorder. (From ref. 1.)

at the lumbosacral joint when the subject was in a standing position. The effects of a corset were varied and unpredictable. External immobilization with either a corset or a brace did not decrease lumbosacral rotation during normal level walking; in fact, these supports caused an increase in the amount of rotation during walking. The average figures for the extent of rotation measured at moderate walking speed (4.6 km/hr) were 1.49° without support, 1.65° with a brace, and 1.63° with a corset.

The effectiveness of external immobilization depends on friction applied to the skin by the corset or brace; therefore the larger the surface area, the greater is the purchase of the external device. The lower part of the thorax presents a relatively wide surface area to which an external device may be applied. In contrast, the surface area available for fixation of the pelvis is much more limited, mainly because, for practical purposes, an external device attempting to grasp the pelvis must not extend so far distally that it prevents hip flexion. For these reasons, motion that normally occurs in the upper lumbar and thoracic spine may be restricted by adequate fixation of these higher levels. Because of relatively poor fixation at the base of the

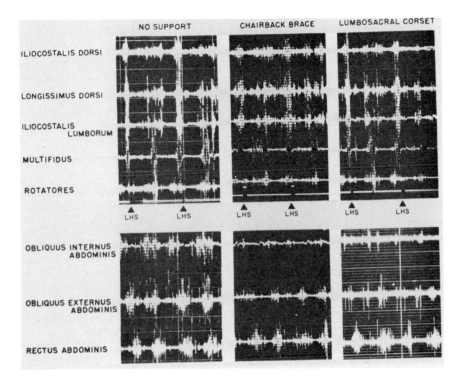

FIG. 4. Records obtained from a subject walking at 5.20 km/hr. LHS — Left heel strike. (From ref. 5.)

appliance or to the pelvic area, rotation that would normally occur in the lumbar spine above the lumbosacral area is diminished, and this motion is transmitted to the lumbosacral level.

Note that in both of the studies the subjects were essentially normal and had no history of significant back pain. It may well be that the effects of an external support are quite different in patients with painful back symptoms.

The effect of spinal supports on electrical activity in the trunk muscles was studied by Waters and Morris (5). When the subjects were standing, the chairback brace and the lumbosacral corset either decreased or had no effect on the electrical activity of the deep back muscles (erectors spinae). When the subjects walked at a comfortable speed, neither support altered the muscle activity significantly. However, when the subjects wore the chairback brace and walked at a fast pace, activity of the back muscles increased in most subjects in comparison with the level of activity when no support or a corset was worn (Fig. 4). It appears that the different effect on electrical activity by the chairback brace and the lumbosacral corset is caused by the brace's more rigid construction. Transverse rotation of the trunk is an inherent feature of ambulation. Wearing a chairback brace or a corset does not significantly alter these rotations; they still occur within the confines of the support. The extent of restriction of the transverse rotation of the trunk by a support depends on its rigidity and the adequacy of its fixation to the trunk. In fact, the increased activity in the back muscles recorded in subjects walking rapidly while wearing the chairback brace must reflect the increased muscular exertion of the back muscles as they attempt to overcome the immobilizing effect of the brace. However, since persons with low back pain do not ordinarily walk rapidly, this finding is presumably of little clinical significance. A flexible lumbosacral corset worn at both fast and slow walking speeds apparently does not exert restrictive forces significant enough to alter muscle effort and electrical activity of the erector spinae muscles.

Both types of support either decreased or had minimal effect on the amount of electrical activity in the abdominal muscles (internal and external obliques), as recorded at rest and during slow walking. The effect on the abdominal muscles is explained by the fact that both the corset and brace have flexible corset fronts and exert forces on the anterior aspect of the trunk during ambulation. Therefore the requirement for muscle activity to support the abdominal contents and maintain intraabdominal pressures is decreased.

If low back supports do not immobilize the spine and do not have a significant effect on the activity of the back muscles, how can they significantly reduce symptoms of low back pain? In order to explain this, it may be of value to review briefly the role of the trunk in the support of the spine.

As noted in the discussion of spinal mechanics, the spine may be considered a segmented elastic column supported by the paraspinal muscles. This column is attached to the sides of, and is situated within, two chambers: the thoracic and abdominal cavities. The thoracic cavity is filled largely with air, and the abdominal cavity with a semifluid mass. The action of the trunk musculature converts these chambers into nearly rigid walled cylinders containing (a) air and liquid, and (b) liquid and solid material. Both of these cylinders are capable of resisting part of the force generated in loading the trunk, thereby relieving the load on the spine itself.

When stress is applied to the spine, there is a reflex increase of intraabdominal pressure. This is a well-known phenomenon. Whenever a heavy weight is to be lifted or pushed, there is a reflex inspiration and tightening of the abdominal musculature. Increase of the pressure by wearing a wide, tightened belt is also a longstanding practice of stevedores and weight lifters. It has also been observed for many years that, in certain cases of low back pain caused by "mechanical instability," or "disc degeneration," compression of the abdominal viscera often relieves the pain. This compression may be accomplished by a circumferential bandage, a well-fitting corset, a brace with an abdominal pad that can be tightened, or a snug plaster body jacket.

Nachemson and Morris (3) studied the effects of wearing a tightened lumbosacral corset on the intradiscal pressures recorded *in vivo*. They found that, when a lumbosacral corset was tightened to the point of tolerance, intradiscal pressure at the base of the lumbar spine could be reduced by up to 30%.

It appears therefore that probably one of the most significant effects of the lumbar supports, including corsets and braces, is compression of the abdomen. It results in increased abdominal pressure, which creates a semirigid cylinder that surrounds the spinal column, and it is capable of relieving some of the stresses imposed on the vertebral column.

CLINICAL USE OF EXTERNAL SUPPORTS

Bracing or support of the spine may be provided for symptoms resulting from trauma (i.e., fractures, infections, and muscle weakness of the intrinsic back or abdominal muscles) and occasionally from metabolic bone disease (e.g., osteoporosis).

The vast majority of supports or braces, however, are prescribed for symptoms arising from degenerative disc disease, either before attempted surgical treatment or after failure of operation to eliminate symptoms. In deciding whether to use a support, it is important to evaluate the stage of degenerative disc disease. Briefly, it can be divided into the following stages:

1. "Acute back pain"
   Early
   Resolving
2. Chronic disc degeneration
   Intermittent acute episodes
   Persisting symptoms due to posterior facet arthritis
   Persisting pain after unsuccessful surgery, with or without pseudarthrosis
3. Acute or chonic symptoms due to disc prolapse or herniation

Treatment of the acute stage of degeneration generally involves bed rest and medication followed by physical therapy—specifically, an abdominal muscle-strengthening program. If the symptoms persist for more than 10–14 days, a support (e.g., a lumbosacral corset) frequently aids in mobilizing the patient. After the symptoms have subsided, an exercise program is again instituted in an attempt to prevent a recurrence.

In the case of chronic disc degeneration with intermittent acute episodes, a support such as a corset or a lumbosacral brace of the chairback type that restricts anteroposterior and mediolateral motion frequently helps the individual to remain active and more comfortable during the acute episode. Again, note that the support is used only as a temporary symptomatic measure and is discontinued as soon as the symptoms have subsided.

In the case of persisting low back pain due to posterior facet arthritis or failure of surgical treatment with or without pseudarthrosis, there are occasional instances in which prolonged and continuous use of the brace or support is necessary to keep the patient functioning. In this instance we found that a light-weight, laminated fiberglass or plastic body jacket with or without inflatable pads at the lower pelvic brim and over the abdomen is of benefit. The cost of such an appliance, however, does not warrant its routine use with acute temporary episodes of low back pain. Even in these cases, the goal should be to wean the patient from the support and allow his own trunk musculature to provide the stability and support for the low back area.

Results from using supports on patients with acute or chronic symptoms due to disc prolapse or herniation are generally disappointing. Frequently the sciatic symptoms are aggravated by the support. Presumably this occurs on the basis of increased blood flow through Batson's plexus as a result of abdominal compression. This increase in blood flow may produce further inflammation and irritation to the damaged nerve root.

SUMMARY

An understanding of what a back support or brace can or cannot do is important. The back support can restrict but not prevent motion in the lower lumbar region. A restrictive support produces primarily abdominal compression, which transforms the abdominal contents into a semirigid cylinder capable of transmitting stresses through the abdomen rather than the vertebral column per se. The use of such a restrictive back support is only a temporary measure. The goal of treatment is restoration of physiological forces that support the spine through the action of the individual's trunk musculature.

REFERENCES

1. Lumsden, R. M., II, and Morris, J. M. (1968): An in vivo study of axial rotation and immobilization at the lumbosacral joint. *J. Bone Joint Surg.,* 50A:1591.
2. Lusskin, R., and Berger, N. (1975): Prescription principles. In: *Atlas of Orthotics: Biomechanical Principles and Application.* Mosby, St. Louis.
3. Nachemson, A., and Morris, J. M. (1964): In vivo measurements of intradiscal pressure: Discometry, a method for the determination of pressure in the lower lumbar discs. *J. Bone Joint Surg.,* 46A:1077.
4. Norton, P. L., and Brown, T. (1957): The immobilizing efficiency of back braces: Their effect on the posture and motion of the lumbosacral spine. *J. Bone Joint Surg.,* 39A:111.
5. Waters, R. L., and Morris, J. M. (1970): Effect of spinal supports on the electrical activity of muscles of the trunk. *J. Bone Joint Surg.,* 52A:51.

Spinal Deformities and Neurological Dysfunction, edited by S. N. Chou and E. L. Seljeskog. Raven Press, New York © 1978.

Neurourological Evaluation in Patients with Neurovesical Dysfunction: Techniques and Pathophysiological Significance

Gaylan L. Rockswold

Department of Neurosurgery, University of Minnesota; and Division of Neurosurgery, Hennepin County Medical Center, Minneapolis, Minnesota 55415

Urinary bladder dysfunction secondary to spinal cord injury and disease is a major source of morbidity and disability (4,22). Neurogenic bladder with its resultant urinary incontinence and malfunction is not only a psychological and social nuisance and embarrassment, but the chronic effects on renal function and general health are often very serious. It is the purpose of this chapter to describe the pathophysiology of neurovesical dysfunction secondary to spinal disease, the techniques used in evaluating this problem, and finally an approach to management based on this evaluation.

EFFECT OF SPINAL INJURY ON MICTURITION REFLEXES

There is considerable evidence that micturition is a brainstem-organized reflex rather than one organized at the sacral level (1,9,16). Neural impulses originating from sensory receptors in the bladder wall travel via the lateral columns of the spinal cord to the reticular formation of the pons (2,6,12,40). Synaptic connections are made in the brainstem; cerebral inhibition is released; and efferent impulses return via the lateral columns of the spinal cord to the anterior horn cells of the detrusor nucleus in the sacral gray matter. A sustained, coordinated detrusor contraction results which is capable of evacuating the intravesical contents. The anatomic integrity of this "long routed" reflex is necessary for an effective detrusor reflex.

Complete interruption of this detrusor reflex pathway produces detrusor areflexia and urinary retention as seen in spinal shock. Over a period of 2 to 6 weeks reflex detrusor function begins to return (25). A recircuiting of the reflex arc distal to the spinal cord injury could occur on the basis of collateral sprouting of dorsal root axons (30,31). This concept is supported by deGroat and Ryalls' (16) experimental work in cats, which showed that the latencies of reflex discharges recorded in parasympathetic neurons evoked by stimulation of the pelvic nerve were much shorter following spinal cord transection than those elicited in the intact spinal cord isolated from supraspinal input.

Partial spinal cord injury frequently results in a low-threshold detrusor reflex which is frequently unsustained and uncoordinated. Unilateral lesions of the spinal cord do not produce significant clinical bladder symptoms due to the extensive crossover in the lumbar area of the descending tracts conducting impulses to the bladder (2,40).

Injury to the conus medullaris, cauda equina, or pelvic nerves results in detrusor areflexia and flaccid sphincters. In this situation either the anterior horn cell or its axon is destroyed, and the opportunity for the development of reflex bladder function does not exist. If the lesion is incomplete in its destruction of neuronal function, however, recovery may be possible.

DIAGNOSTIC METHODS AND FINDINGS

Gas Cystometry

The basic neurourological diagnostic procedure is cystometry. This consists of retrograde filling of the urinary bladder through an indwelling catheter with either gas or liquid with constant recording of intravesical pressure. Carbon dioxide has been preferred over saline because of much faster filling times and less artifact related to the decreased viscosity of air (5). There is no more than a 10% decrease in volumes recorded owing to the compressibility of CO_2 compared to saline at the intravesical pressures recorded (14).

The principal observation made from the cystometrogram is the presence or absence of a detrusor reflex (37). The reflex stimulus is passive distention of the bladder, and the response is a contraction of the detrusor muscle producing an intravesical pressure rise. If a detrusor reflex is evoked, the patient is asked to suppress the reflex as a test of detrusor reflex volitional control. Inability to suppress the reflex is an event frequently termed an uninhibited detrusor reflex (Fig. 1). Since this often occurs with a low-

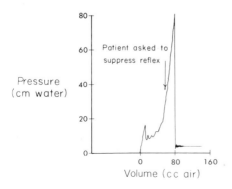

FIG. 1. Cystometrogram demonstrating detrusor hyperreflexia.

volume reflex threshold, it has been termed detrusor hyperreflexia. Clinically, these cystometrogram findings were associated with the sensation of urgency and frequently precipitate voiding with little voluntary control. This syndrome can develop from incomplete lesions of the spinal cord secondary to trauma, arachnoiditis, congenital deformities, and tumors. Detrusor hyperreflexia can also develop following a complete transverse spinal cord lesion above the conus medullaris. This occurs with the development of reflex bladder function dependent on the distal spinal cord.

Complete absence of a detrusor reflex is termed detrusor areflexia (Fig. 2). This diagnosis can be made only with caution, since suppression of the detrusor reflex can result from the embarrassment or discomfort of the examination situation. Areflexia can also result from various nonneurological causes, e.g., chronic catheter drainage, urinary infection, and overdistention of the bladder. Various drugs including the phenothiazines, belladonna derivatives, and ganglionic blocking agents can also produce detrusor areflexia. It is important to rule out the presence of obstruction in the lower urinary tract in these cases.

Patients with the syndrome of detrusor areflexia most frequently relate a history of difficulty initiating voiding and not infrequently of complete retention. If voiding does occur, the flow rate is frequently decreased and

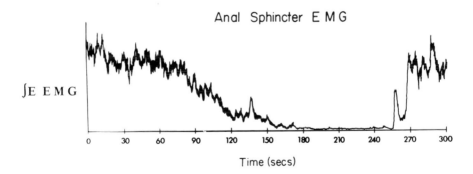

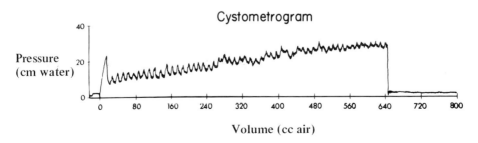

FIG. 2. Detrusor areflexia associated with uninhibited sphincter relaxation with increasing bladder distention.

intermittent with a significant residual urine present. Various neurologic disorders can produce detrusor areflexia, including traumatic injury to the cauda equina or conus medullaris; the stage of spinal shock following injury to the supranuclear portion of the spinal cord; centrally located herniated lumbar discs; arachnoiditis of the cauda equina; spinal cord birth defects, most prominently myelomeningocele; and tumors of the conus medullaris and/or cauda equina.

Anal and Urethral Sphincter Electromyography

Anal sphincter electrical activity is studied with the aid of an anal plug with bipolar externally mounted recording electrodes (8). A bipolar concentric recording electrode is also mounted on a urethral catheter in order to study urethral sphincter activity. This electrode design obviates the discomfort and inconvenience of the insertion and reinsertion of needle electrodes. The net electrical output of the sphincter is measured in contrast to the localized sample recorded by needle electrodes. Patients are asked to contract the sphincters volitionally to determine if supraspinal innervation is intact.

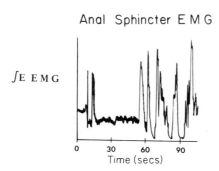

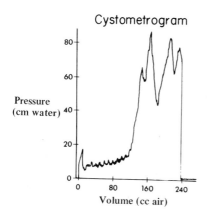

FIG. 3. Detrusor hyperreflexia with detrusor–sphincter dyssynergia.

dence of hydronephrosis, hypoplastic kidney, ureteral reflux, and other abnormalities associated with chronic neurogenic bladder disease.

Urologic Consultation

In the evaluation of any neurologic bladder disease, close cooperation with a urologist who is familiar and interested in this problem is obviously beneficial and at times essential. Treatment of upper urinary tract complications including calculosis, hydronephrosis, pyelonephritis, ureteral reflux, as well as lower urinary tract obstruction fall clearly within the domain of the urologist.

TREATMENT OF DETRUSOR HYPERREFLEXIA

The goal of treating hyperreflexia is to reduce the hyperactivity of the detrusor muscle so that the bladder can tolerate larger volumes of urine without the symptoms of frequency and urgency. At the same time, effective voiding should be maintained without the accumulation of significant residual urine.

Drugs

An initial trial of drug therapy is indicated in patients suffering from detrusor hyperreflexia. Methantheline bromide (Banthine) is perhaps the initial drug of choice. Methantheline is a synthetic anticholinergic compound which blocks the postganglionic synapses at the usual doses used (24). The usual dose is 50 up to 100 mg q.i.d. A closely related compound, propantheline bromide (Pro-Banthine), can also be used in doses of approximately 15 mg q.i.d. Various antiganglionic agents (e.g., mecamylamine hydrochloride; Inversine) which produce autonomic ganglionic blockade can also be used in the treatment of detrusor hyperreflexia (42). A significant problem with these agents has been the hypotension produced. Each of the agents has a tendency to produce increased residual urine as well as side effects (e.g., constipation and blurring of vision) caused by blocking of the autonomic system at unwanted sites. In summary, these agents appear worth an initial trial in the case of detrusor hyperreflexia. The main difficulties include the close proximity of the therapeutic dose to doses producing unacceptable side effects and ineffective voiding with increased residual urine.

Sacral Nerve Block

Selective sacral nerve block can be carried out in certain patients to determine which of the sacral nerves is operative in detrusor reflex activity (35).

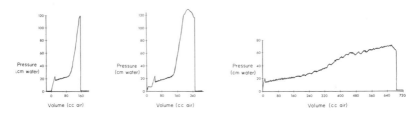

FIG. 5. Effect of sacral nerve blocks on the cystometrogram. **Left:** Control cystometrogram showing low threshold detrusor hyperreflexia. **Center:** Cystometrogram following a unilateral S3 block showing little change. **Right:** Cystometrogram following unilateral S3 and S4 blocks showing absence of detrusor reflex and significant increase in bladder capacity.

By sequentially blocking several of the sacral nerves with local anesthesia using cystometric control, the detrusor reflex can be abolished and bladder capacity significantly increased (Fig. 5). In essence, this method determines the functional innervation of the detrusor muscle by determining which sacral nerves are primarily operative in detrusor reflex function. In a series of 50 patients so studied, we determined that the detrusor reflex could be abolished with unilateral sacral block in approximately 50% (35). Anesthetizing only two sacral nerves ipsilaterally produced this effect in 17 patients. In this situation one can then consider either more permanent sacral blocks with the use of phenol or possibly a radiothermal lesion. This usually provides relief of symptoms for 3 to 12 months. Possible complications include a painful neuritis resulting from intraneural injection of the phenol. Advantages include the fact that a surgical procedure is avoided and the block can be quite easily repeated in the case of recurrent symptoms.

Sacral Rhizotomy

If detrusor hyperreflexia can be reduced and bladder capacity increased by anesthetizing two or three sacral nerves, the patient can be considered a candidate for selective differential sacral rhizotomy (34,36). Using the operating microscope, the individual fascicles of the selected sacral roots can be, in turn, stimulated and anesthetized to identify fibers which innervate the bladder only. These can then be sectioned, leaving the remainder of the nerve intact. Thus more physiologic voiding can be restored for the patient by preserving the detrusor reflex and sphincter function but at the same time increasing bladder capacity. There has been no difficulty postoperatively with disturbance in sexual function in the patients treated. The primary difficulty has been in recurrent symptoms over a period of long-term follow-up. Thus in a group of 13 patients so treated only 6 remained symptomatically improved for over 2 years. However, there was no morbidity or mortality in this group of patients.

TREATMENT OF DETRUSOR AREFLEXIA

Drugs

Treatment of patients with detrusor areflexia should be directed toward achieving satisfactory emptying of the urinary bladder. Drugs again are worth an initial trial in the management of this problem. Bethanechol chloride is probably the most frequently used and most useful drug for this purpose. Bethanechol is an analog of acetylcholine which has a reasonably selective action on the gastrointestinal (GI) tract and urinary bladder (26). The side effects include increased salivation, sweating, intestinal cramps, and diarrhea. Neostigmine (Prostigmin) is a synthetic anticholinesterase drug. It is sometimes useful where bethanechol is not effective, but in general it is not used as commonly. It is absorbed rather poorly from the GI tract and also probably has a direct stimulator effect chronically on denervated skeletal muscle and sympathetic ganglia (26).

Intermittent Catheterization

Intermittent catheterization can be an effective way of treating detrusor areflexia with secondary inability to empty the urinary bladder. It has been most extensively used in paraplegic and quadriplegic patients during the period of spinal "shock" to aid in emptying the bladder and to restore automatic or reflex bladder emptying. Sir Ludwig Guttman (20) introduced the technique of intermittent catheterization for paraplegics following the second World War. His reports clearly document its value in rendering the patient catheter-free with a significantly decreased incidence of infected urine. The complications of the indwelling Foley catheter—which include hydronephrosis, vesicle-ureteral reflux, renal and/or vesicle calculi, fistulas, prostatitis, seminal vesiculitis, and epididymitis—are clearly decreased. However, it has only been with considerable delay and seeming reluctance that physicians in the United States have begun to accept the value of this technique (3,21). However, more recently there are several authors who again clearly demonstrated the value of intermittent catheterization following spinal cord injury (3,17,29,33).

Ideally intermittent catheterization should begin shortly after the injury so that an indwelling Foley catheter is never inserted. However, numerous authors have shown that intermittent catheterization may start several weeks or even months later and be of value in rendering the patient catheter-free and in clearing infection. The patient is catheterized using aseptic techniques approximately every 4 to 6 hr initially. Prior to catheterization attempts are made to promote reflex emptying of the bladder, e.g., stroking the inner thigh, manipulation of the anal sphincter, or squeezing the glans. As bladder function begins and some emptying of urine occurs, the catheterizations are spaced from the initial 4 hr to 6, 8, 12, and 24 hr according to the residual urine. Thereafter catheterization is done every 48 or 72 hr, or once weekly, depending on bladder function before it is abandoned completely. Urecholine in doses of 5 to 50 mg q.i.d. are effective in inducing the return of bladder tone and efficient detrusor contraction. The routine use of methenamine mandelate (Mandelamine) 1 g and ascorbic acid 1 g q.i.d. is recommended as a urinary suppressant.

The fact that patients can be made catheter-free following spinal cord injury with intermittent catheterization is related to the fact bladder filling represents the physiologic stimulus for micturition by setting up appropriate afferent impulses to the spinal cord. Although there is no direct neurophysiologic proof for this concept, it is known that continuous bladder drainage reduces detrusor excitability and its ability to contract effectively to artificial stimulation in animals (18). In addition, the continuous distention of the external urethral sphincter by the cannula provides another source of unbalanced reflex activity between the detrusor muscle and the pelvic floor muscles. The absence of infection would also contribute to the earlier return of bladder reflex function.

Using this technique, the vast majority of patients can be rendered catheter-free. In one controlled prospective study, two groups of 50 patients each were compared (29). There were follow-up studies of up to 5 years on each group. One group was treated by the traditional method of an indwelling Foley catheter removed for trials of voiding and the second group by intermittent catheterization. Only 18 of 50 patients became catheter-free using the traditional techniques of an indwelling Foley catheter removed on several occasions for trials of voiding. All of the patients treated with intermittent catheterization became catheter-free 1 to 6 months after injury (average 3 months). Intermittent catheterization was carried out for a period of 2 to 70 days (average 11 days). The incidence of urinary infection, urinary calculi, and deterioration of renal function clearly showed the intermittent catheterization treatment to be superior. It seems conclusive that intermittent catheterization is the treatment of choice for patients with detrusor areflexia following spinal cord injury.

Intermittent catheterization is also useful in other diseases producing detrusor areflexia. Patients who have undergone laminectomy for various intraspinal lesions with a period of prolonged postoperative detrusor areflexia can be treated with intermittent catheterization. Recovery of spontaneous voiding is enhanced. If detrusor areflexia persists, the patient can be taught the technique of self-intermittent catheterization (27,32). Patients have found this technique quite satisfactory over long periods of time. Objections concerning the introduction of an infection may be raised. However, it has been shown that indwelling urinary catheters are perhaps the greatest source of infection (15). The bladder has an inherent resistance to infection in the absence of a foreign body. In the presence of an indwelling Foley catheter, virtually all patients with neurologic bladder problems become infected within a few days. Patients using clean self-intermittent catheterization have fewer infections than those with chronic indwelling catheters. Also the various other complications of the indwelling catheter previously mentioned are avoided.

Detrusor Stimulation

Considerable effort has been put into stimulating the detrusor muscle electronically to achieve effective urinary bladder evacuation (10). However, great difficulty has been encountered in rendering this a consistently effective technique. The single most important problem has been the inability to couple electrical energy effectively to stimulate contraction of the smooth muscle cells of the detrusor muscle. The cellular arrangement for spread of excitation in the detrusor muscle is such that two-thirds to three-fourths of the surface area of the detrusor muscle must be directly activated by electrical stimulation to produce effective evacuation. In addition, the electrodes which cover such a large surface area must be sufficiently flexible to maintain contact with the bladder wall during the contour changes that occur during the course of bladder emptying. At the present time detrusor stimulation appears to be an experimental technique which holds promise and should be continued at certain centers.

Sacral Cord Stimulation

In a few centers evacuation of the bladder contents is produced by placing chronic stimulating electrodes in the sacral spinal cord of spinal cord injury patients (19). This procedure has been carried out only in patients who are completely paraplegic and in whom attempts at training a reflex bladder have been completely unsuccessful. The primary problem with this technique has been to obtain selective stimulation of the detrusor muscle only. Stimulation of the intermediolateral cell columns at the S1–S2 levels have produced contraction of the external urethral sphincter via the pudendal nerve, causing outflow obstruction. In several patients this was improved with sphincterotomy. In addition, stimulation of other autonomic pathways produces erection, defecation, and hypotension. The authors reporting on this technique state that these side effects can be reduced by proper stimulus parameters.

Grimes and Nashold (19) reported a series of 10 patients, 6 of whom completely rely on the bladder stimulator for purposes of micturition. All of these patients have remained totally continent of urine and maintain residual urine volumes of less than 10 cc. Their incidence of infection has been markedly reduced. This technique seems promising. The indications for spinal cord stimulation appear to be limited at the present time to complete spinal cord lesions with complete paraplegia, and limited to those few patients in whom adequate reflex bladder function cannot be obtained with intermittent catheterization and other rehabilitative measures.

TREATMENT OF SPHINCTER DYSFUNCTION

Persistent detrusor-sphincter dyssynergia producing ineffective bladder emptying and/or persistent vesicoureteral reflux and hydronephrosis can be satisfactorily treated with external sphincterotomy (23). Ephedrine sulfate can be used effectively to increase the tone of the bladder outlet in cases of uninhibited sphincter relaxation. This effect is probably secondary to the dense sympathetic innervation of the bladder neck and proximal urethra (7). A prosthetic urinary sphincter can be used in situations of complete denervation of the sphincter (39).

SUMMARY

Evaluation and management of neurogenic bladder disease remains a very difficult and occasionally baffling problem. The above outline of a diagnostic and therapeutic approach is by necessity oversimplified. However, it is hoped that by a systematic and multidisciplinary approach our understanding of the complexities involved, and thereby our therapeutic attempts, will be improved.

REFERENCES

1. Barrington, E. J. F. (1921): The relation of the hindbrain to micturition. *Brain,* 44:23–52.
2. Barrington, E. J. F. (1933): The localization of the paths subserving micturition in the spinal cord of the cat. *Brain,* 56:126–148.
3. Bors, E. (1967): Intermittent catheterization in paraplegic patients. *Urol. Int.,* 22:236–249.
4. Boyarsky, S., editor (1967): *Neurogenic Bladder.* University Park Press, Baltimore.
5. Bradley, W. E., Clarren, S., Shapiro, R., and Wolfson, J. (1968): Air cystometry. *J. Urol.,* 100:451–455.
6. Bradley, W. E., and Conway, C. J. (1966): Bladder representation in the pontine-mesencephalic reticular formation. *Exp. Neurol.,* 16:237–249.
7. Bradley, W. E., Rockswold, G. L., Timm, G. W., and Scott, F. B. (1976): Neurology of micturition. *J. Urol.,* 115:481–486.
8. Bradley, W. E., Scott, F. B., and Timm, G. W. (1974): Sphincter electromyography. *Urol. Clin. North Am.,* 1:69–80.
9. Bradley, W. E., and Teague, C. T. (1968): Spinal cord organization of micturition reflex afferents. *Exp. Neurol.,* 22:504–516.
10. Bradley, W. E., Timm, G. W., and Chou, S. N. (1971): A decade of experience with electronic stimulation of the micturition reflex. *Urol. Int.,* 26:283–303.
11. Bradley, W. E., Timm, G. W., Rockswold, G. L., and Scott, F. B. (1975): Detrusor and urethral electromyelography. *J. Urol.,* 114:891–894.
12. Bradley, W. E., Timm, G. W., and Scott, F. B. (1974): Innervation of the detrusor muscle and urethra. *Urol. Clin. North Am.,* 1:3–27.
13. Cardus, D., Quesada, E. M., and Scott, F. B. (1963): Studies on the dynamics of the bladder. *J. Urol.,* 9:425.

14. Cass, A. S., Ward, B. D., and Marklund, C. (1970): Comparison of slow and rapid fill cystometry using liquid and air. *J. Urol.,* 104:104–106.
15. Cox, C. E., and Hinman, F. (1965): Retention catheterization and the bladder defense mechanism. *JAMA,* 191:105–108.
16. DeGroat, W. C., and Ryall, R. W. (1969): Reflexes to sacral parasympathetic neurones concerned with micturition in the cat. *J. Physiol. (Lond.),* 200:87–108.
17. Firlit, C. B., Canning, J. R., Lloyd, F. A., Cross, R. R., and Brewer, R. (1975): Experience with intermittent catheterization in chronic spinal cord injury patients. *J. Urol.,* 114:234–236.
18. Geise, A., Bradley, W., Chou, S., and French, L. (1963): Effect of indwelling catheter on electrical excitability of the bladder. *Surg. Forum,* 14:493–494.
19. Grimes, J. H., and Nashold, B. S. (1974): Clinical application of electronic bladder stimulation in paraplegics. *Br. J. Urol.,* 46:653–657.
20. Guttman, L. (1954): Statistical survey on one thousand paraplegics and initial treatment of traumatic paraplegia. *Proc. R. Soc. Med.,* 47:1099–1109.
21. Guttman, L., and Frankel, H. (1968): The value of intermittent catheterization in the early management of traumatic paraplegia and tetraplegia. *Paraplegia,* 5:63–84.
22. Hald, T. (1969): Neurogenic dysfunction of the urinary bladder: An experimental and clinical study with special reference to the ability of electrical stimulation to establish voluntary micturition. *Dan. Med. Bull. (Suppl. V),* 16:1–156.
23. Herr, H. W., Engelman, E. R., and Martin, D. C. (1975): External sphincterotomy in traumatic and non-traumatic neurogenic bladder dysfunction. *J. Urol.,* 113:32–34.
24. Innes, I. R., and Nickerson, M. (1975): Atropine, scopolamine, and related antimuscarinic drugs. In: *The Pharmacological Basis of Therapeutics,* edited by L. L. Goodman and A. Gilman. Macmillan, New York.
25. Jonas, U., Jones, L. W., and Tanagho, E. A. (1975): Recovery of bladder function after spinal cord transection. *J. Urol.,* 113:626–628.
26. Koelle, G. B. (1975): Parasympathomimetic agents. In: *The Pharmacological Basis of Therapeutics,* edited by L. L. Goodman and A. Gilman. Macmillan, New York.
27. Lapides, J., Diokno, A. C., Silber, S. J., and Lowe, B. S. (1971): Clean, intermittent self-catheterization in the treatment of urinary tract disease. *Trans. Am. Assoc. Genitourin. Surg.,* 63:92–95.
28. Lapides, J., Friend, C. R., Ajemian, E. P., and Reus, W. C. (1962): Denervation supersensitivity as a test for neurogenic bladder. *Surg. Gynecol. Obstet.,* 114:241–244.
29. Lindan, R., and Bellomy, V. (1975): Effect of delayed intermittent catheterization on kidney function in spinal cord injury patients; a long-term follow-up study. *Paraplegia,* 13:49–55.
30. Liu, C. N., and Chambers, W. W. (1958): Intraspinal sprouting of dorsal root axons; development of new collaterals and preterminals following partial denervation of the spinal cord in the cat. *Arch. Neurol. Psychiatry,* 79:46–61.
31. McCough, G. P., Austin, G. M., Liu, C. N., and Liu, C. V. (1958): Sprouting as a cause of spasticity. *J. Neurophysiol.,* 21:205–216.
32. Orikasa, S., Koyanagi, T., Motomura, M., Kudo, T., Togashi, M., and Tsuji, I. (1976): Experience with non-sterile, intermittent self-catheterization. *J. Urol.,* 115:141–142.
33. Perkash, I. (1975): Intermittent catheterization and bladder rehabilitation in spinal cord injury patients. *J. Urol.,* 114:230–233.
34. Rockswold, G. L., Bradley, W. E., and Chou, S. N. (1973): Differential sacral rhizotomy in the treatment of neurogenic bladder dysfunction. *J. Neurosurg.,* 38:748–754.
35. Rockswold, G. L., Bradley, W. E., and Chou, S. N. (1974): Effect of sacral nerve blocks on the function of the urinary bladder in humans. *J. Neurosurg.,* 40:83–89.
36. Rockswold, G. L., Bradley, W. E., and Chou, S. N. (1974): Differential sacral rhizotomy. *Minn. Med.,* 57:586.
37. Rockswold, G. L., Bradley, W. E., Timm, G. W., and Chou, S. N. (1976): Neurologic bladder dysfunction; evaluation and treatment at the University of Minnesota. *Minn. Med.,* 59:687–691.
38. Rockswold, G. L., Bradley, W. E., Timm, G. W., and Chou, S. N. (1976): Electrophysiological technique for evaluating lesions of the conus medullaris and cauda equina. *J. Neurosurg.,* 45:321–326.

39. Scott, F. B., Bradley, W. E., and Timm, G. W. (1974): Treatment of urinary incontinence by an implantable prosthetic urinary sphincter. *J. Urol.,* 112:75–80.
40. Stewart, C. C. (1899): On the course of impulses to and from the cat's bladder. *Am. J. Physiol.,* 2:182–202.
41. Susset, J. G., Picker, P., Kretz, M., and Jorest, R. (1973): Critical evaluation of uroflow-meters and analysis of normal curves. *J. Urol.,* 109:874–878.
42. Volle, R. L., and Koelle, G. B. (1975): Ganglionic stimulating and blocking agents. In: *The Pharmacological Basis of Therapeutics,* edited by L. L. Goodman and A. Gilman. Macmillan, New York.

Spinal Deformities and Neurological
Dysfunction, edited by S. N. Chou and
E. L. Seljeskog. Raven Press, New York
© 1978.

Spinal Cord Injury and Cost Accounting: A Preliminary Report

Theodore M. Cole

Department of Physical Medicine and Rehabilitation, University of Minnesota
Medical School, Minneapolis, Minnesota 55455

Spinal cord injury with paralysis almost always elicits feelings of hope-lessness and foreboding. The first recorded reference to the injured spinal cord was found in the Edwin Smith Surgical Papyrus (6) written 2500 to 3000 B.C. "Thou shouldst say concerning him, one having a dislocation of the vertebra of his neck while he is unconscious of his two legs and two arms and his urine dribbles, an ailment not to be treated." Almost five millennia later in his novel *All the King's Men*, Robert Penn Warren described the quadriplegic life as one of helplessness, hopelessness, and impending death.

World War I greatly added to the number of patients with spinal cord injuries, and the medical attitude of hopelessness persisted. In his review of the literature, Dick (5) pointed out that until World War II paraplegic patients were neither able nor encouraged to be independent in self-care. The general attitude of hopelessness led many to become addicted to nar-cotics, and the few that survived did so as pathetic wrecks, dependent and helpless, needing care in homes or hospitals for the chonically ill.

During recent years a basic change in the approach to spinal cord injury care has begun to emerge, the roots of which can be found in this country and abroad (2,4,9,14). Several factors contributed to the change in the United States. Most notable was the increasing pressure exerted by the consumer of spinal cord health services—the paraplegic or quadriplegic himself. Working through such national organizations as the Paralyzed Veterans of America and the National Paraplegia Foundation, thousands of paralyzed people succeeded in calling attention to some of the elements of acute and rehabilitative care they believed important. For many, these services made the difference between a successful adjustment to residual disability and a lifetime of medical complications and psychosocial failures. Further, they helped convince the government to undertake research and demonstration projects to test the hypothesis that comprehensive systems rather than fragmented nonsystems of spinal cord injury care yield better outcomes at lower costs. Crisis-oriented care with either strictly medical or vocational objectives came under fire.

Pressures for change were also building from the fiscal intermediaries, private and public. The Liberty Mutual Insurance Company (7) has supported efforts to understand better the problems associated with spinal cord injury. It has also supported research to solve problems through preventive and therapeutic techniques.

Spurred on by Carter (3), Young (16), and Wilcox et al. (15), the Department of Health, Education and Welfare became interested in encouraging systems of spinal cord care and measuring the cost and outcomes of systematic versus nonsystematic care on a nationwide basis. Carter's figures were sobering. Although the national estimated annual mortality of 1,800 to 3,000 cases of spinal cord injury falls well below that of stroke, for example, the annualized estimate of $2.4 billion for spinal cord injury care far outstripped the cost for treatment of the commoner neurological impairments such as stroke, epilepsy, multiple sclerosis, and Parkinson's disease. He showed that the estimated medical expenses of an individual case of traumatic paraplegia at age 29.5 years with a normal life expectancy of 41.4 years was $65,089. The economic cost of traumatic paraplegia over a lifetime was in excess of $300,000.

The impact of the high cost is compounded when one considers that, even after it is paid, neither the patient nor society is benefited by a cure. The disability persists; and in the case of the typical young male patient with a high spinal cord injury, virtually every organ system in the body remains affected for a lifetime. Clearly, a re-examination of spinal cord injury care was in order.

SPINAL CORD INJURY CENTERS

Under support from the Rehabilitation Services Administration, Department of Health, Education and Welfare, a national network of Spinal Cord Injury Centers is now established to demonstrate, within defined regions in the country, a multidiscipline system of comprehensive services extending from the time of detection and evacuation of the injured, through acute care and rehabilitation management, to community and job placement, and long-term follow-up.

There are 11 systems (Table 1), all charged with providing integrated services from the surgical and physiatric disciplines, acute and rehabilitation nursing, vocational counseling, psychology, physical therapy, occupational therapy, social service, and others as needed.

Each system must be able to provide detection and evacuation services that can travel to the location of the injury and transport the patient to a medical facility for emergency evaluation. Whether the patient is transported to a local facility or a regional center depends on his medical status and ability to tolerate travel. It is assumed that well-trained emergency

TABLE 1. *Consortium of spinal cord injury centers*

ALABAMA	**MINNESOTA**
University of Alabama	University of Minnesota Hospitals
Birmingham, Alabama	Minneapolis, Minnesota
ARIZONA	**NEW YORK**
Good Samaritan Hospital	Institute of Rehabilitation Medicine
Phoenix, Arizona	New York, New York
CALIFORNIA	**TEXAS**
Santa Clara Valley Medical Center	Texas Institute of Rehabilitation and
San Jose, California	Research
COLORADO	Houston, Texas
Craig Rehabilitation Center	**VIRGINIA**
Englewood, Colorado	Woodrow Wilson Rehabilitation Center
ILLINOIS	Fishersville, Virginia
Northwestern Memorial Hospital	**WASHINGTON**
Rehabilitation Institute of Chicago	University of Washington Hospital
Chicago, Illinois	Seattle, Washington
MASSACHUSETTS	
University Hospital	
Boston University Medical Center	
Boston, Massachusetts	

medical services personnel are available to make transfer of the patient as safe as possible.

Following emergency evaluation, he is jointly evaluated by specialists in neurosurgery, orthopedics, urology, and rehabilitation who seek to stabilize the medical–surgical problems. During this period of consultation and communication, other members of the spinal cord injury team see the family and the patient, as appropriate. They set into motion a tentative plan for long-range goals and prepare the rehabilitation staff and the patient to work with each other. Issues which may not become paramount until some time in the future are anticipated even at this early date, and resources are identified for later use.

Following medical and surgical stabilization, intensive rehabilitation commences. The focus of care becomes less on medical need and more on self-care, mobility, and psychosocial and vocational–educational issues. The entire rehabilitation process can be regarded as an educational effort directed by a physician, utilizing all members of the spinal cord injury team, and aimed at training the patient and his family to cope effectively with disability in an environment of maximum independence.

Discharge from the hospital, whether to an independent or supportive living situation, does not end the spinal cord team's involvement. Since the disability is often permanent, so too is the need for follow-up. Para-plegics and quadriplegics are not rehabilitated in the sense that they achieve an optimum level of function and stay there. The nature of their disability places them at an increased risk of medical, psychological, social, or voca-tional deterioration, making lifelong enlightened follow-up desirable.

NEUROLOGICAL LEVEL AND FUNCTION

A patient's outcome depends in large measure on the level at which the spinal cord is injured. Most clinicians (10,11) recognize seven critical levels of spinal cord injury. Beginning with the 4th cervical segment, the addition of each successive critical segment adds an important increment to the muscle power of the patient. The quadriplegic who retains the 4th cervical segment continues to have function in the sternomastoids, upper cervical paraspinal muscles, and trapezius muscles. Voluntary use of the arms, trunk, and lower extremities are absent, but he may benefit from training in the use of externally powered devices to substitute for the function of the arms. He can control his head position, which in turn assists in balancing the trunk while sitting in the wheelchair. Many such patients find an adaptive tool held in the mouth for typing, writing, page-turning, etc. to be more useful than adaptive devices attached to the denervated arms.

When the 5th cervical segment is preserved, the deltoid and biceps muscles continue to function, as do the external rotators of the shoulder. These muscles usually remain weak, however, and frequently require external assistance in order to accomplish useful work. The patient lacks elbow, forearm, and hand control, making it necessary to continue use of assistive devices if he is to engage in useful upper-extremity activity. He may be able to do some self-feeding and grooming and to assist in dressing activities. However, he is unable to manually push his wheelchair and requires a motorized wheelchair. He is also unable to assist in transferring himself to or from a chair, bed, and toilet.

When the 6th cervical segment is retained, the patient may gain some voluntary strength in the shoulder depressors, the scapula stabilizers and shoulder adductors, internal rotators, and radial wrist extensors. These muscles enhance the ability to perform activities of daily living. The wrist extensor mechanism is especially important. It can be harnessed through a special tenodesis splint, which drives the fingers into flexion. He is more capable of pushing his wheelchair if the wheels have adaptive devices to allow his hands to grasp the rims. With training he can often learn to lean on his arms and periodically shift weight off his buttocks, thus increasing his sitting tolerance to 6 to 8 hr. He can be useful in dressing himself and assisting others in transferring him from bed to chair, etc. Some patients with 6th cervical segment function intact are able to operate safely an automobile with special adaptive equipment.

When the 7th cervical segment is retained, the patient gains some voluntary control over his elbow extensors. Wrist and finger extension may become stronger, and he may gain some use of his finger flexors. He is now able to do pushups on the arms of his wheelchair, and therefore his sitting tolerance can be expected to increase to the limit of his overall physical endurance. Most importantly, hand function is sufficient to allow him to grasp and release voluntarily. This adds important control over activities of daily living as well as greatly increasing his potential for vocational activity. He is thus independent in his wheelchair and should need no motorized assistance. With training he can harness his hand control to irrigate his catheter or stimulate his rectum for bowel movement.

When the lesion is at the upper thoracic level, the patient has full control of his upper extremities and is therefore more properly called paraplegic than quadriplegic. He is completely independent in his wheelchair. With motivation and skills, he is able to work full time and can live independently in a community that has no major architectural barriers to his wheelchair. He is independent in managing his urinary drainage apparatus and in inserting rectal suppositories or a gloved finger for stool extraction.

The next critical level is the lower thoracic or upper lumbar segments. This paraplegic has full abdominal, upper back, and respiratory control. He can do all the activities listed above and more. Because of his increased trunk innervation, his sitting balance is improved, allowing him greater capabilities for wheelchair operation, althletics, and other skills.

When the lower lumbar spinal cord is transected, the patient may retain the use of his hip flexors and knee extensors. However, voluntary control over hip extensors and abductors may be lacking. He may be able to walk with proper bracing and training, but the energy required for functional ambulation is so high as to make it necessary for many such patients to retain the use of a wheelchair on certain occasions.

DATA COLLECTION SYSTEM

The spinal cord centers listed earlier are cooperating in a broad data collection system. The information they collect is biographical, medical, psycho-social-sexual, and vocational-educational. Information is also collected relating to mobility and self-care. The data items themselves have been selected on the basis of collectability, reliability, and meaningfulness.

One set of data reflects the time interval between the onset of spinal cord injury and discharge from comprehensive rehabilitation. Another set is collected on each anniversary of the spinal cord injury. The information is gathered from the spinal cord injury system hospital and from all other hospitals and health care professionals from whom the patient has received care. Additional information is gathered from community agencies and from the patient himself. Examples of issues being addressed are: (a) costs of spinal cord injury, both human and economic; (b) preventative maintenance services; and (c) efficiency of a system approach to treatment. In addition, similar data will be gathered on approximately 500 patients from other nonsystem hospitals, rehabilitation centers, and insurance companies. This information will serve as a comparison to the data collected from system hospitals. Cost effectiveness conclusions can then be drawn.

The system hospitals are also attempting to separate system from non-system patients. System patients are defined as those who receive the full impact of systematized care from the time of the traumatic event and remain in the system throughout follow-up. Nonsystem patients are those who enter the system hospital at some time other than immediately after the traumatic event, who leave the system before completion of their rehabilitation, or who elect not to be followed by the system hospital.

HOSPITALIZATION DATA

Only preliminary information is available from this collaborative study. Tabulation included in the remainder of this report comes from the Southwest Regional System for Treatment of Spinal Injury and the National Spinal Cord Injury Data Research Center, Phoenix, Arizona (8); the Midwest Regional Spinal Cord Injury Care System, Northwestern University, Chicago, Illinois (13); and the Regional Spinal Cord Injury System, University of Minnesota, Minneapolis, Minnesota.

The mean age of onset of spinal cord injury is 31 years. Some centers are experiencing a bimodal curve with a peak in the 16 to 25-year age group and another in the 31 to 35-year age group. At Northwestern Memorial Hospital in Chicago, where the Illinois State Trauma System has a highly developed subsystem for evacuating patients, 65% of the patients were admitted less than 9 hr after their injury in 1975. Twenty percent were admitted during the first week after injury, and the remaining 15% were admitted less than 1 month after injury.

The percentage of quadriplegic and paraplegic patients varies from one center to another. During 1970 to 1971 the Southwest Regional System's inpatients numbered 27.2% quadriplegics and 72.8% paraplegics. In 1975 at Northwestern Memorial Hospital, 53% of the patients were quadriplegics and 47% paraplegics. During the first 10 months of 1976 at the University of Minnesota, 59% of the spinal cord injured patients were quadriplegics and 41% paraplegics.

The percentage of patients who die during the first few weeks varies from center to center and seems to fall as each center gains more experience. In 1971 Phoenix reported a 10% early death rate. Northwestern has experienced a 7% early death rate overall since 1972; and for the first 10 months of 1976 Minnesota reported a 2% early death rate.

The length of stay in the hospital following spinal cord injury has dropped dramatically during the last 25 years. In 1950 it was common for a patient to be hospitalized for 1 year after injury. By 1960, 240 days was typical; and by 1970, 150 days. For the first 10 months of this year, the University of Minnesota found that system quadriplegics remain in the hospital an average of 54 days and nonsystem quadriplegics an average of 94 days. System paraplegics remain in the hospital 52 days and nonsystem paraplegics 84 days. Although these data suggest continued progress toward shortening the period of hospitalization, a wait-and-see attitude is necessary to determine if patients discharged within such a short period fare well during the subsequent years of follow-up. Certainly these preliminary data suggest that the average time from injury to home may be shortened to perhaps 3–4 months. However, long-term adjustment, family education, bladder training, etc. cannot be accomplished in all patients in such a short time. Subsequent short hospitalizations may be preferable for achieving these goals while at the same time allowing time away from the hospital for integration of the need to learn with available services for training. It therefore appears that not only arc we learning how to shorten the duration of hospitalization but we are also shortening the duration of hospitalization for system patients more than we are for those who do not receive systematized care.

The complications of spinal cord injury are myriad. Among the most common are skin pressure ulcers and urinary tract infections. Over the years 1973 to 1975 at the Midwest Regional Spinal Cord Injury Care System in Chicago, a difference was found between the prevalence of decubitus ulcers in system patients as compared to nonsystem patients: Decubitus ulcers developed in 29% of system patients but in 56% of nonsystem patients. With regard to urinary tract infections, virtually all patients treated at Northwestern Memorial Hospital in 1975 developed urinary tract infections: 92% of the system patients and 88% of the nonsystem patients. Considering the expense of these complications, their reduction would greatly reduce the overall cost and improve the health of patients.

Measures of physical function are made during hospitalization and the follow-up period as well. The Barthel index measures independence in individual subtasks of mobility and activities of daily living. The maximum score is 100 units for the patient who is entirely independent in these tasks. At Northwestern Memorial Hospital in 1975, the average spinal cord-injured patient was admitted with a score of 26. At discharge his function had increased to 58 units, and at the end of 1 year postinjury it was 71 units for 98 patients. Although the system patients were 5 units higher at discharge and 2 units higher at the 1-year follow-up than the nonsystem patients, these differences are probably not significant.

VOCATIONAL-EDUCATION PLACEMENT DATA

Postdischarge vocational-education placement of the spinal cord-injured patient has been of great concern to society, which ultimately must accept the cost of reduced productivity. In 1975, 200 vocationally aged, eligible spinal cord-injured patients came into the vocational rehabilitation unit of the spinal cord injury center at Northwestern Memorial Hospital. Of these, 134 cases have been closed, with 67% being placed, although not all gainfully. Of those placed, 29% were gainfully placed and went to work (59% to college, high school, or vocational training programs), 10% are functioning homemakers, and 2% are in sheltered workshops. The number of persons gainfully placed increases with the time following discharge. The Midwest Regional Spinal Cord Injury System followed its patients from earlier years and concluded that maximum placement level is not reached even at 2 to 3 years after injury. By the fourth year following injury, 67% of the patients were gainfully placed; by the third year 46%; and during the first year 21%. This pattern implies a long-term placement process and shows the benefits of aggressive vocational follow-up.

KIDNEY FOLLOW-UP DATA

There is an almost infinite number of parameters one could analyze in the late follow-up of the spinal cord-injured patients. This chapter focuses on only a few. One of the major medical concerns in the long-term management of spinal injuries is renal function. Price et al. (12) conducted an ongoing project to study renal function in patients with spinal cord injury. During the eighth year of her 10-year continuing study, she reported that 78% of patients had good function, 13% mild deterioration, and only 4% moderate deterioration. Five percent had severe deterioration of kidney function. Her studies are based on glomerular filtration rate, renal plasma flow, and maximal tubular excretory capacity using inulin and sodium hippurate clearances and tubular saturation with p-aminohippuric acid (PAH). These data stand in sharp contrast to the expectations of only 30 years ago when renal deterioration was thought to be the primary cause for late demise in spinal-injured people. Price found that the duration of the spinal cord lesion appeared to have little influence on renal deterioration. She also found bladder drainage difficult to assess since all patients had at some time or another used an indwelling catheter and had had accompanying bacteriuria. Factors which did appear to be predictive in renal function assessment were vesicoureteral reflux demonstrated by cystoureterography, kidney stones, blunting of the caliceal pattern as observed by intravenous pyelography, and the development of multiple decubiti.

SOCIAL ADJUSTMENT DATA

The lightening bolt-like change in the body's motor and sensory function following spinal cord injury is so devastating that most patients must invest a great deal of energy and receive much assistance in achieving a satisfactory adjustment for themselves and their families. An insight into the need for counseling is seen by reviewing some of the outcomes that a representative group of adults with paralysis can anticipate. The following are data selected from studies by Athelstan (1) at the Research and Training Center,

University of Minnesota and continued at the Regional Spinal Cord Injury Center. A total of 256 patients from 2 to 22 years postinjury responded to questionnaires to provide data on their status. The age and sex distribution and the levels of injury were representative for a typical population of spinal cord-injured adults. Approximately four out of five were males, and the modal age group was below 30 years. Approximately half were paraplegics and the other half quadriplegics. An examination of these data provides a realistic framework for the future following discharge from the hospital. These expectations in turn can serve as guidelines for the physician who is answering the patient's questions about the future. The counseling process is, of course, the bridge between the present, the patient's expectations, and realities of life in the future (Figs. 1–4).

Social adjustment can be understood in part by examining marital and dating status, living arrangements, and frequency of getting out of the home. Figure 1 shows that less than half of this group of former patients are married. Slightly more of them date members of the opposite sex, with slightly over a third dating with any frequency. With respect to living arrangements, 18% are living either in a nursing home or receiving care from an attendant; 37% are living with a spouse; and 25% have returned to their

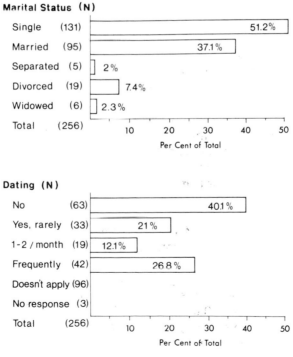

FIG. 1. Follow-up psycho-social-vocational data on 256 patients questioned 2–22 years after spinal cord injury: marital status and dating. (From ref. 1.)

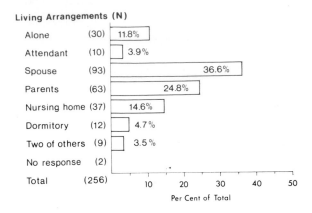

FIG. 2. Follow-up psycho-social-vocational data on 256 patients questioned 2–22 years after spinal cord injury: living arrangements and frequency of getting away from home. (From ref. 1.)

parent's home. Only 12% are living alone. A measure of social adjustment as opposed to social withdrawal is the frequency with which the former patient gets out of the home. Almost two-thirds venture out at least once a week, which suggests that they are continuing to interact socially with their environment. One-third are getting out rarely or less than once a week, and it is this group who are probably experiencing moderate to severe social withdrawal (Fig. 2).

Athelstan found that only 44% of the women and 39% of the men in his group reported themselves as working. In Fig. 3, the annual income and reasons given by the nonworkers for not working are analyzed. Two-thirds of the former patients are earning an income below a level which would be considered adequate for the average person. However, approximately 16% are earning greater than $10,000 a year. Of those who do not work, physical limitation is the reason given by 35% of them. This, coupled with 11% who give medical problems as reasons for not working, suggest that almost half of the unemployed former patients attribute their reason for not working to the spinal cord injury.

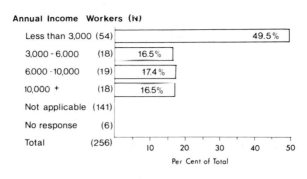

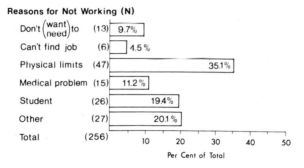

FIG. 3. Follow-up psycho-social-vocational data on 256 patients questioned 2–22 years after spinal cord injury: annual income of workers and reasons for not working. (From ref. 1.)

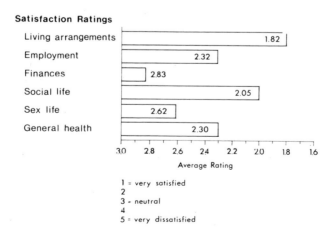

FIG. 4. Follow-up psycho-social-vocational data on 256 patients questioned 2–22 years after spinal cord injury: satisfaction ratings. (From ref. 1.)

Lastly, an overall rating of patient satisfaction is seen in Fig. 4. Not surprisingly, the patient's financial situation is the least satisfactory aspect of his life following spinal cord injury. Also interestingly, sex life is listed as the second most dissatisfied area studied. Both of these measures fell below the neutral point in the satisfaction-dissatisfaction scale.

COST DATA

Ultimately, the cost of all benefits, complications, and treatments must be measured to determine cost effectiveness. The National Spinal Cord Injury Data Research Center in Phoenix, Arizona, has been collecting and storing data submitted by the consortium of 11 spinal cord injury systems. Although these data are only in the earliest stages of assembly, a preliminary look is of interest.

Table 2 breaks out the cost data on a combined population of paraplegics and quadriplegics for three variables during initial spinal cord injury system hospitalization and seven variables during a typical anniversary year after the injury. The data represent information gathered on system patients only and compare the combined experience of the consortium of 11 centers with the experience of the Minnesota center alone. The Minnesota data are for the first anniversary year, which is an average of 10 months. It should be noted that median figures, shown in $500 increments, are used rather than mean figures. This was done because the mean value was often inflated

TABLE 2. *Selected cost data on system paraplegic and quadriplegic patients*

Variable	Eleven centers combined		Minnesota only	
	No. of patients	Median cost ($)	No. of patients	Median cost ($)
Initial SCI system hospitalization				
Hospitalization expense	222	14,750	36	11,750
Physician fees	109	1,250	33	1,250
Equipment expense	191	750	38	250
Subtotal		16,750		13,250
Anniversary year				
Hospitalization expense	81	500	12	1,000
Physician fees	42	500	12	500
Outpatient therapies	47	500	12	500
Outpatient medications and supplies	35	500	11	500
Attendant care expenses	76	500	11	500
Custodial care expenses	77	500	12	500
Vocational rehabilitation expenses	59	500	12	500
Subtotal		3,500		4,000
Total		20,250		17,250

with high costs sustained by a comparatively small number of patients. Only actual dollar figures were used. No estimates were accepted.

It can be seen that on a national average the combined median cost of the three variables listed during the initial spinal cord injury hospitalization is $16,750. Additional expenses incurred during the first anniversary year add $3,500 to this figure, giving a total of $20,250 as a median cost for the year following spinal cord injury. The Minnesota experience is only slightly different. The combined median cost of the three variables during the initial spinal cord injury system is $13,250. To this is added $4,000 of cost incurred during the first anniversary year, yielding a grand total of $17,250. These costs might be anticipated for the average paraplegic-quadriplegic over the course of 1 year after spinal cord injury.

THE SURGEON AS FACILITATOR

The neurosurgeon or orthopedic surgeon who has first contact with the newly spinal cord-injured patient is in a unique position to initiate the complex interactions of the comprehensive treatment program. He is also in a position to help the patient and patient's family understand and begin to accept the fact of the spinal cord injury and the need to look beyond the immediate medical and surgical problems to the lifetime of education and training that are necessary to cope with the chronic disability.

The surgeon can aid the patient by projecting a positive yet realistic attitude toward the disability. To the extent that the surgeon deals directly with the sequelae of spinal cord injury, the patient is positively encouraged to begin the process of self-reassessment that leads to the necessary changes. If the surgeon avoids a direct and informative approach, no matter how sensitive the subject area, the patient may begin construction of defense barriers to protect himself from the psychological impact of the injury. Later, removal of these barriers by the rehabilitation staff often requires extensive work. Sometimes the barriers cannot be removed. It has been our experience that patients benefit from being fully informed about their neurological prognosis and the medical and surgical procedures which may be necessary. They also benefit from being encouraged to deal with the disability forthrightly with their own families.

The surgeon is usually in charge of the patient immediately after injury. He can also help the patient by making it possible for the multidisciplined spinal cord injury team to have its effect. This means that most spinal cord-injured patients should be seen immediately by physicians from other specialities, e.g., rehabilitation medicine, urological surgery, and when necessary respiratory medicine, general surgery, and internal medicine. The patient should also be evaluated immediately by physical and occupational therapists, a counseling psychologist, a social worker, and a vocational rehabilitation counselor. These people bring to the patient the foundations for the broad education necessary for an optimum outcome. Provisions must also be made for these professionals to interact with other members of the spinal cord injury team including the physicians. In this way, a uniform presentation is made, and the patient is receiving consistent messages. Not to do this is to risk individual interpretations by each member of the team, with the patient being caught in the middle of mixed and sometimes conflicting information. All of this should be started as soon as the patient is medically and surgically stable.

Later, when the patient leaves the acute surgical area and begins rehabilitation, it is vital that the surgeon continue to follow him. This provides continuity of physician services, which the patient needs. It also assures the rehabilitation team of the continued expert opinion of the surgeon in the aftercare of fracture and spinal instability.

The surgeon is responsible during the time when decisions are made that deal with life and death and partial or complete recovery of neurological function. However, this period in the patient's evolution as a paraplegic or quadriplegic is extremely short when compared with the lifelong process of adjustment and education. The surgeon does well to remember that the major therapeutic mode which soon will benefit the patient is educational and not medical or surgical. The timely relinquishing of responsibilities for care to those whose skills and interests lie in this area is one of the hallmarks of the complete surgeon.

ACKNOWLEDGMENT

This project was supported in part by Social Rehabilitation Services Research and Demonstration Grants 13-P-55916 and 13-P-55258, and by Minnesota Medical Rehabilitation Research and Training Center No. 2 Grant 16-P-56810.

REFERENCES

1. Athelstan, G. (1975): Ongoing research project reported in annual report of Minnesota Medical Rehabilitation Research and Training Center, No. 2. University of Minnesota, Minneapolis.
2. Bedbrook, G. M. (1967): The organization of a spinal injuries unit at Royal Perth Hospital. *Paraplegia,* 5:150–158.
3. Carter, R. E. (1972): Research and training center accomplishments in spinal cord injury. Presented at the Conference of Rehabilitation, Research and Training Centers, Temple University, Philadelphia.
4. Cheshire, D. J. E. (1968): The complete and centralized treatment of paraplegia. *Paraplegia,* 6:59–73.
5. Dick, T. B. S. (1969): Traumatic paraplegia pre-Guttmann. *Paraplegia,* 7:173–177.
6. Elsberg, C. A. (1931): The Edwin Smith Surgical Papyrus and the diagnosis and treatment of injuries to the skull and spine 5000 years ago. *Ann. Med. Hist.,* 3:271–279.
7. Freed, M. M., Bakst, H. J., and Barrie, D. L. (1969): Life expectancy, survival rate, and causes of death in civilian patients with spinal cord trauma. *Arch. Phys. Med. Rehabil.,* 47:457–463.

8. Grant Progress Report (1972): SRS Grant No. RD337-M-70. Good Samaritan Hospital, Phoenix, Ariz.
9. Guttmann, Sir L. (1967): History of the national spinal injury services, Stoke Mandeville Hospital, Aylesbury. *Int. J. Para.,* 5:115–126.
10. Long, C. (1971): Congenital and traumatic lesions of the spinal cord. In: *Handbook of Physical Medicine and Rehabilitation,* edited by F. H. Krusen, F. J. Kottke, and P. M. Ellwood, Jr., pp. 566–578. Saunders, Philadelphia.
11. Long, C., and Lawton, E. B. (1955): Functional significance of spinal cord lesion level. *Arch. Phys. Med. Rehabil.,* 36:249–255.
12. Price, M., Kottke, F. J., and Olson, M. E. (1975): Renal function in patients with spinal cord injury: The eighth year of a ten-year continuing study. *Arch. Phys. Med. Rehabil.,* 56:76–79.
13. Progress Report IV (1975–1976). Grant No. 13P-55864. Northwestern Memorial Hospital (Wesley Pavillion) and Rehabilitation Institute of Chicago.
14. Weiss, M. (1967): 15 Years experience on rehabilitation of paraplegics at the Rehabilitation Institute of Warsaw University, Poland. *Paraplegia,* 5:1158–1166.
15. Wilcox, N. E., Stauffer, E. S., and Nickel, V. L. (1970): A statistical analysis of 423 consecutive patients admitted to the spinal cord injury center, Rancho Los Amigos Hospital, 1 January 1964 through 31 December 1967. *Paraplegia,* 8:27–35.
16. Young, J. S. (1976): United States National Spinal Cord Injury Data Research Center. *Paraplegia,* 14:81–86.

Subject Index

Abnormalities; *see also* specific name
  developmental, of spinal cord, 41–51
  of vertebral column, 41–51
Achondroplasia, cervical involvement of, 94
  clinical findings in, 82–94
  head size and, 95
  low back pain and, 95
  neurological symptoms, 82, 92–94
  radiographic findings, 75–82, *76–81*
  scoliosis and, 95
  spinal surgery and, 83–91
  symptoms, 82–94
Anal sphincter electromyography, 244, 245
Anatomy, of spine, 25, 26
Anomaly(ies), vertebral, 46–51; *see also*
  specific name
Anoxia, spinal blood supply and, 17, 18
Anterior interbody fusion, spondylolithesis
  and, 195
Anterior neuropore, formation of, 3
Anterior spinal cord syndrome, 71
Anulus, force-deflection curve and, *29*, 30
Arch, neural, nonsegmentation of elements,
  48, 49
Areflexia, detrusor, *see* Detrusor areflexia
Arteries, spinal, 11–14, *12*, *13*
Arthritis, achondroplasia and, 79
  rheumatoid, basilar erosion and, *115*
Axial load
  cervical spine injuries and, 67, *68*
  lumbar spine injuries and, 69
Axial rotation
  intervertebral joint and, 30–32, *31*, *32*
  of spine, *in vivo*, 32–34, *33*, *34*

Back bracing, consequences, 231, 232
Basilar coarctation, 114
Basilar erosion, 114, 115, *115*
Bending, intervertebral joint and, 30
Biomechanics, of intervertebral joint, 27, 28
Blood circulation, spinal cord, collateral,
  18–20
  physiology of, 17–21
Blood, spinal cord, clinical problems and,
  18–20
Bone, spine fusion and
  cancellous, 147
  cortical, 147, 148
  grafts, 147, 148
Braces; *see also* Supports
  design of, 232, 233

Bracing, low back, consequences of, 231,
  232
Brain, formation of, 3
Brown-Sequard syndrome, 71

Canalization, 4, *4*, 5
Cancellous bone, spine fusion and, 147
Capener procedure, description of, 132
  steps in, *133*
Carcinoma, metastatic, 116, *116*
Catheterization, intermittent, in detrusor
  areflexia, 249–251
Central spinal cord injury syndrome, 71
Cervical spine
  deformity of, with neurologic dysfunction,
    113–129
  fusion of, indications for, 148
    techniques for, 149, *149*, *150*, *151*
  injuries to, mechanism of, 66–68
  lower, deformities in, 123–129
  mid, deformities in, 123–129
  upper, deformities in, 113–123
Children, paraplegia in, 167–171, *168–171*
Chondrification, in formation of vertebral
  column, 8, *8*
Circulation, of blood, *see* Blood circulation
Claudication, intermittent, achondroplasia
  and, 82
Clinical problems, collateral blood circula-
  tion and, 18–20
Collateral blood circulation, in spinal cord,
  18–20
Cortical bone, spine fusion and, 147, 148
Cost data, spinal cord injury and, 266, 267
Creep, intervertebral disc and, 29
Curvature, of spine, myelographic evalua-
  tion of, 99–111
Cystometry, gas, in neurovesical dysfunc-
  tion, 242–244
Cystourethrogram, use of, 246, 247

Deformity(ies), of cervical spine, with
  neurologic dysfunction, 113–129
  following laminectomy, *see* Postlamin-
    ectomy kyphosis
  in lower cervical spine, 123–129
  in mid cervical spine, 123–129
  progressive, with stable spine, 113–117,
    123–125
  with spinal instability, 117–123, 125–129

271

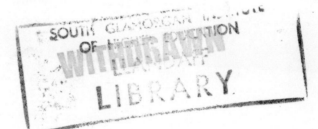